I0082778

Gastric Sleeve Cookbook

A Food Guide to Stages One and Two of Your Gastric Sleeve Surgery Recuperation

© **Copyright 2016 by John Carter - All rights reserved.**

This document is geared towards providing exact and reliable information in regard to the topic and issue covered. The publication is sold with the idea that the publisher is not required to render accounting, officially permitted, or otherwise, qualified services. If advice is necessary, legal or professional, a practiced individual in the profession should be ordered.

- From a Declaration of Principles which was accepted and approved equally by a Committee of the American Bar Association and a Committee of Publishers and Associations.

In no way is it legal to reproduce, duplicate, or transmit any part of this document in either electronic means or in printed format. Recording of this publication is strictly prohibited and any storage of this document is not allowed unless with written permission from the publisher. All rights reserved.

The information provided herein is stated to be truthful and consistent, in that any liability, in terms of inattention or otherwise, by any usage or abuse of any policies, processes, or directions contained within is the solitary and utter responsibility of the recipient reader. Under no circumstances will any legal responsibility or blame be held against the publisher for any reparation, damages, or monetary loss due to the information herein, either directly or indirectly.

Respective authors own all copyrights not held by the publisher.

The information herein is offered for informational purposes solely, and is universal as so. The presentation of the information is without contract or any type of guarantee assurance.

The trademarks that are used are without any consent, and the publication of the trademark is without permission or backing by the trademark owner. All trademarks and brands within this book are for clarifying purposes only and are the owned by the owners themselves, not affiliated with this document.

Bonus:

FREE Report Reveals The Secrets To Lose Weight

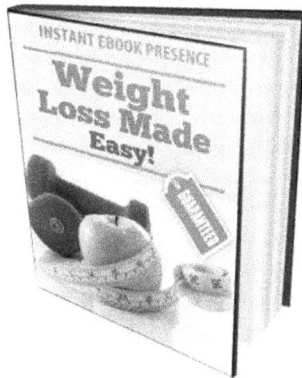

Weight loss doesn't happen from dieting only. Diets are short term solutions to shed extra weight. Diets do not work in the long term because people hate being on a diet (it's ok, you can admit that here). The only long term solution for permanent weight loss is to create new eating habits. This doesn't mean that chocolate will never pass your lips again, but it does mean looking after yourself and watching what you eat...

You can lose weight when you have the right reasons and motivation, and a part of this guide is to help you to find the motivation you need to change your weight...

Go to Get This Guide For FREE

http://www.sportsforsoul.com/weight-loss-2/

Table of Contents

Introduction

I want to thank you and congratulate you for downloading the book, *"Gastric Sleeve Cookbook: A Food Guide to Stages One and Two of Your Gastric Sleeve Surgery Recuperation."*

While your doctor likely gave you some suggestions for what to eat or sent you to his dietitian, you can use this book to explore additional recipes. This book contains proven steps, strategies and blender recipes for creating tasty meals that will best enable a gastric sleeve patient to recuperate.

You've just lost part of your stomach and now you need to figure out tasty menu options that you can have in small amounts for the next several weeks. You also need to be sure that you get sufficient nutrition from much less food than you are used to eating, though you will also need to take supplements now and for the rest of your life.

You won't feel well during those first few weeks after your surgery, so you won't want to spend a lot of time in the kitchen. Yet, you need to feed yourself nutritious and good-tasting meals and drinks.

We understand. You will find strategies in this book that will help you to get through this difficult time with as little trouble as possible. You will also discover many recipes for easy-to-make, tasty and nutritious smoothies and shakes, along with ideas for some soft food combinations that will help you on your journey back to good health. You will, no doubt, continue to make some of the delicious smoothies and shakes after you have recuperated!

Thanks again for downloading this book. I hope you enjoy it!

Chapter 1:
Steps and Strategies for Success

Before Your Surgery

If you have not yet had your surgery, there are some things you can do ahead of time that will help you during those painful days.

- **Change your diet.**
You need to prepare your body for this procedure by going on a high-protein liquid diet one or two weeks before your surgery. This will shrink your liver, making the surgery safer for you.

- **Change your grocery list.**
You need to have a lot of protein-rich liquids before surgery and after surgery. Clear liquids are what you will consume immediately after your surgery for a day or two. After that phase, you will advance to protein shakes and pureed food.

- **Get the clothes you will need.**
You will need transition clothes for the various weights that you will be. You will want your initial clothing after the surgery to fit loosely. You will also want slip-on shoes so that you won't have to bend over to tie your shoes.

- **Stop smoking.**
Surgeons take smoking seriously. Just before surgery, they will likely give you a blood test to see whether you have been smoking lately. If you have, they will cancel your surgery. Why? If you are smoke-free, your recovery will be quicker. You will need to quit smoking one month before your surgery.

- **Pack your hospital bag.**

You will stay at the hospital one night, so pack whatever you will need for one night.

- **Prepare your support group.**

You will need both physical and mental support after your surgery. You need to educate people before your surgery and line volunteers up who can help you while you recover.

- **Get your insurance or other financing source ready.**

Your health insurance may not pay for this kind of surgery. Typically, body mass index and other health issues are involved. Get the financials ready to pay for your surgery.

- **Get ahead of the household chores and shopping before surgery.**

Make lots of smoothies (minus the ice cubes), cook and freeze meals, clean the house, and do all of the laundry before you go in for surgery so that nobody has to do those things later. Buy the stool softeners, over-the-counter medications and your prescriptions (if possible) ahead of time.

Your friends and family may help you, but it would be easier for everyone if you have most of the work done ahead of time. You will also be certain to not lack for anything while you are at a disadvantage.

- **Get the facts.**

Talk to your surgeon about any concerns or questions you have about your surgery so that you have a good understanding about what will be done and be less anxious about your surgery.

- **Study up on proteins.**

You will need to consume a lot of protein after your surgery. You need to try protein powders to discover which ones you like among the ones that won't add a lot of calories. Food sources are peanut butter, legumes, chicken, meats, and protein shakes.

After Your Surgery

- **Follow your doctor's prescribed diet.**

Eat what your doctor tells you to eat after your surgery, which will consist of a lot of liquid. If you eat regular food too early or if you eat sugary or fat food, you may damage your stomach or harm yourself.

- **Skip work until you have healed.**

Depending on which kind of surgery you have and what type of work you do, you could be back to work as soon as two weeks after surgery if you do not lift anything heavy.

- **Exercise when you can.**

Wait about four weeks before you exercise or lift weights so that you will decrease the chance that you will get a hernia in the wound.

- **Go to your check-ups.**

Let your doctor check on your progress at the scheduled times. He'll see whether or not you are on schedule in your weight loss goals.

- **Continue to find suitable foods you can eat.**

You need to try out new recipes so that you can stay on your diet plan. You don't want boredom with your food to turn you back to your old eating habits.

- **Take multivitamins.**

It will be hard to get all of the nutrition that you need from just your food, especially less food, so be sure to take a multivitamin daily.

- **Know when to ask for help.**

Right after your surgery, it will be hard to get anything done. Hopefully, you got your chores done, groceries and meds purchased, food pre-made and frozen, and your helpers lined up before you went into surgery. Don't be afraid to call on the friends and family who agreed to help you when you need them, especially if you notice a complication.

- **Follow your prescription.**

Keep taking your prescribed medication for as long as you were supposed to take it. Don't get off of it early. Make an appointment with your doctor if you have discomfort beyond what is normal.

- **Count the calories.**

If you keep your calorie intake between 600 and 800 per day, you will lose weight. Consult your doctor for his suggested calorie target. Don't eat high-calorie food, especially those with sugar and/or fat.

- **Don't drink your calories.**

Drink water, unsweetened ice tea, and sugar-free juice. You will need to use up your daily allotment of calories on food that contains protein instead of drinks with "empty calories."

Chapter 2:
What Can I Eat?

What to Eat for the First 30 Days after Surgery

Stage One

Food and Drink Choices

You need to follow your doctor's orders as far as when, how much, and what foods you can consume after your gastric sleeve surgery. However, this guide can give you an idea of what to expect.

Surgery day – The staff will put you on intravenous fluid, but you will have to drink about one fluid ounce of water (and only water) per hour. You will be given one-ounce medicine cups to measure out and sip your water from, and you will be required to make notes regarding your water intake.

Day One - Usually by noon on the day following your surgery, you will start to consume between one and three ounces of broth, sugar-free gelatin, decarbonized ("flat") diet ginger ale, or water per hour.

You will need to stop drinking as soon as you feel full. Don't force yourself to drink more than you are comfortable drinking. However, the goal will be for you to reach a drinking capacity of one quart (32 ounces) per day. You will likely reach that goal within that day. Once you do, the intravenous fluids can be discontinued.

Day Two - Usually by the second day out from your surgery, you will take in low-sugar, enriched liquids. You will do this for *two to three weeks*.

You will take in four fluid ounces of a nutritional supplement every other hour over and eight-hour period per day. Between these supplements, you will drink between four and eight fluid ounces of various clear liquids.

These liquids include the following:
- decaffeinated herbal tea
- decaffeinated coffee
- fruit juice (no added sugar, max 4 ounces per serving and 8 ounces daily)
- sugar-free popsicles (under 20 calories, up to two daily)
- tomato juice
- V-8 juice
- flat diet decaffeinated soda
- broth
- sugar-free drinks like Kool-Aid or Crystal Light
- water.

Fluid goal: The fluid goal is for you to reach a capacity of six cups of liquid per day of both the nutrient-enriched beverage and the clear liquids. Stop when full, though, and don't push things beyond what is comfortable.

Protein goal: You will need to consume at least 70 grams of protein per day, which is usually what is in seven scoops of protein powder. You will need to track your protein intake.
Supplements: Take these with your meals. You will need to take two multivitamins in chewable form in addition to three 600 mg of calcium carbonate and vitamin D in chewable form daily.

Reminders: Take 30 minutes to sip your liquids and continue to record all food and fluid intake.

Stage Two

Two to Three Weeks Out – Two or three weeks after your surgery, you can gradually introduce pureed and soft food that resembles the consistency of applesauce and up to a very soft consistency.

You will consume thick liquids, such as protein shakes and pureed food, using your blender for most of what you consume during this phase. Because of their high protein content, the protein shakes will be useful to you on days when you are having trouble reaching your daily intake of protein.

You won't be using a straw (because it might introduce air to your stomach), but the food will need to be blended so small that it could fit through a straw.

Your pureed food will resemble baby food. In fact, you can eat baby food, but only the pureed meat ones contain the protein you need. You will likely enjoy pureed meat that you make yourself better, though.

You may not be able to tolerate meat until later on in this stage. You can see how you do with meat later on if you want to. There are many other tasty choices available that will give you the protein and other nutrients you need.

You need to have six meals per day and take the supplements and liquids in between meal times, not with the meals. Remember to chew well all food that needs to be chewed.

Chapter 3:
Soft/Pureed Food Cooking Tips and Menu Ideas for Your Stage Two Diet

You'll want to ease into this stage consuming things like Lactaid-free milk, almond milk, unsweetened coconut milk, blended Greek yogurt with no fruit chunks, unsweetened applesauce, cooked cereal such as oatmeal, grits or Cream of Wheat made with lactose-free milk, blended soup made with lactose-free milk, blended fruit smoothies and shakes.

Do not combine food selections below right at first in any one meal, but gradually try the following foods during this phase:

Light white fish
Crackers with peanut butter
Cooked eggs
Cooked vegetables
Soft fruit
Yogurt with fruit
Cottage cheese
Oatmeal, grits or Cream of Wheat
Blended soup

You may tolerate meat, however, so you can test your tolerance and see. After all, you won't want to only consume breakfast food and sweet-tasting shakes for longer than you have to.

Below, you can find sources of protein and also food from the various food groups that you ought to begin to consume during this phase.

Protein Sources

Protein is essential for our bodies to function properly, and you need to concentrate on consuming liquid protein when you first get out of your surgery. Protein will speed up the healing process, enhance your fat burning metabolism, and minimize your hair loss.

Besides a deficiency in protein, hair loss is also associated with a deficiency in iron and zinc, so you'll need to make sure you take multivitamins. You will likely lose some hair anyway about a half year after your surgery for a little bit, so you will want to be sure that you give it all of the nutrients that you can to eventually come out of this experience thin, with muscle tone and a full head of hair.

Eat lots of protein and take your vitamins! You'll need to take in around 70 grams of protein per day during this phase.

Remember that you will need to mash or puree foods that are not already soft. Here are some good sources of protein:

Protein Source Grams per Serving	Serving Size	
Protein powders (for smoothies)	1 scoop	20-40
Cooked vegetables	.5 cup	1-2
Instant breakfast drinks	1 packet	4-15
Tofu	3 oz.	11
Soy veggie burger	1	9

Bread	1 slice	2
Rice	.5 cup	5
Noodles/macaroni	.5 cup	3-4
Dry cereal	1 oz.	5
Oatmeal	1 cup	5
Nuts	.25 cup	4.5
Lima beans	.5 cup	5
Peanut butter	2 T	8.5
Beans: brown, kidney, black-eyed peas garbanzo, white, pinto, black	.5 cup	7.5
Fat-free refried beans	.5 cup	8
Reduced fat ricotta cheese	1 oz.	6
Low-fat yogurt	1 cup	8-12
Non-fat milk powder	1 T	2.5
Skim milk/1% milk	1 cup	8
Low-fat cottage cheese	.5 cup	13
Egg substitute	.25 cup	6
Egg whites	2 T	9
Egg	1 med	7
Lean meat: pork, beef, fish, chicken	1 oz.	7

Other sources of protein include:

- Nonfat dry milk powder (Add this to hot cereals, soups, casseroles, etc.)
- Legumes
- Fish
- Cream of Wheat with skim milk
- Strained cream soups, such as chicken, mushroom, potato or celery
- Baby food meats
- White fish, such as orange roughy, tilapia, haddock and cod
- Canned chicken breast
- Canned tuna in water

Grains and Starches

You will need to mash or puree foods that are not already soft. Good sources of grains and starches include the following:

- Winter squash
- Mashed potatoes
- Sweet potatoes
- Baby oatmeal
- Grits
- Farina

Fruit

You will need to mash or puree foods that are not already soft. Good sources of fruit include the following:

- Peaches
- Apricots
- Melons
- Pineapples
- Pears
- Bananas
- Canned fruit in own juices
- Applesauce
- Juice sweetened with a non-nutritive sweetener
- Diluted 100% apple juice
- Diluted 100% grape juice
- Diluted 100% cranberry juice

Vegetables

You will need to mash or puree foods that are not already soft. Good sources of vegetables include the following:

- Diet V-8 Splash
- V-8 Juice
- Other tomato juice
- Spinach
- Green beans
- Summer squash
- Carrots

Note: Avoid cauliflower, broccoli or other fibrous veggies during your stage two, pureed food time.

Drinks
Make sure that you consume at least eight cups of low-calorie, caffeine-free liquids throughout the day so that you will prevent yourself from becoming dehydrated.

Sip these drinks *between the meals.* Do not drink with the meals. Wait for 30 to 45 minutes after you finish your meal before you drink fluids.

The following items are examples of drinks you can have:
- Sugar-free flavored drinks
- Skim milk
- Decaffeinated coffee (maximum 8 ounces per day)
- Decaffeinated tea (maximum 8 ounces per day)
- Diet fruit drinks (under 10 calories per day)
- Water
- Sugar-free flavored water
- Zero-calorie flavored water

Supplements
You will also need to start taking supplements daily that contain the following:
- Iron
- Zinc
- Calcium citrate
- B12
- Other supplements as indicated from your lab results

Take them in chewable form for the first month (something like Flintstones) twice daily. You can start taking vitamins and minerals in pill form after your first post-operative month if you prefer pills.

Lactose and Food Intolerances

Some gastric sleeve patients become intolerant to lactose after their surgery, so you'll need to use unsweetened coconut milk, almond milk, or Lactaid-free milk.

If you have pain or vomit after you introduce a new kind of food, go back to your liquid diet for an entire day before trying pureed food again. Don't let it discourage you. Notate when you ate the problem food, what food it was that gave you the problem, and what your reaction was to it.

You may not be able to tolerate poultry or other meat for a while after your surgery. If you have trouble tolerating some of the pureed meat, you might want to wait until later in this phase to try meat. You can just label it and freeze it.

Alternatively, you can introduce meat in small amounts, blended in with potatoes or other vegetables and/or sauces. There are recipes for meat dishes in this book that you can make. Many of them are various veggie-rich meatball and sauce meals that you eat in blended form while you are in the early stages after your gastric sleeve surgery.

Food to Avoid

Sugar and carbs can easily sabotage your weight loss efforts, as can bad fats or even good fats if eaten excess. Avoid the following foods to prevent sabotaging your weight loss efforts:

- Fried food
- Doughnuts
- Alcohol
- Ice cream
- Sherbet
- Preserves

- Cakes
- Molasses
- Flavored drink mix
- Honey
- Regular sodas
- Sweets
- Candy

Tips for the First Month after Your Operation

1. Keep food records. You may want to do this indefinitely, just to stay on top of what you're eating, but be sure to do it for that first after your surgery. Notate the following:
   - Time you ate
   - Type of food you ate
   - Amount of food you ate
   - How you prepared your food, including any oils used
   - Protein gram amount wherever you can find this information

2. Use ice trays to control portion size, noting that each cube holds about two ounces. These are good for use with pureed meats and vegetables, low-fat cream soups, etc.

3. Eat only two to four ounces of food per meal, concentrating on protein intake. Try to get 80 grams of protein daily, which protein shakes and supplements would help you to achieve in addition to what you can eat.

4. Try to eat between four and six small meals daily.

5. Take your time eating and drinking. Take half an hour to eat and drink just four ounces, which is half a cup.

6. Drink at least eight cups of liquids daily between the meals, waiting 30 to 45 minutes after your last meal to drink.

Low-fat Cooking Tips

When you get to where you can eat more solid food, prepare the food items as normal and then just puree/blend or mash them. See how you like the taste.

If you don't tolerate meat by itself, you may tolerate a little of it if it is mixed with mashed potatoes, along with low-fat sour cream, or eaten in blended recipe form (See the blended meat recipes).

Poultry and other meat
1. Use lean meat.
    - Top round beef (It's best to forego red meat, however)
    - Turkey, no skin, white meat
    - Chicken, no skin, white meat

2. Trim off the fat.

3. Use low-fat cooking methods.
    - Broil, grill, bake, saute, stir-fry using broth, vegetable spray, small amount of oil, or water

4. Drain off fat.

Vegetables
1. Use "I Can't Believe It's Not Butter" spray for butter flavor without the calories.

2. Add tomatoes, carrots, green peppers and other fresh vegetables to your spaghetti sauces.

3. Add fat-free sour cream or low-fat cottage cheese to potatoes.

4. Cook using methods that do not require fat, such as microwave, steam, grill and bake.

5. Don't cook with bacon, butter or fatback.

6. Avoid high-fat sauces, such as butter, oil, cheese, and sauces made with cream.

Soups
1. Let your soup cool. Skim fat off after it has cooled, accumulated on the top and hardened.

Desserts
1. Use Splenda to add sweetness to smoothies, shakes, unsweetened decaffeinated tea, etc.

2. Read food labels. Only consider food items that have low sugar content or use artificial sweetener.

Modify Recipes
1. Omit unnecessary high-fat ingredients.
   Examples: Oil, cheese, excessive meat, nuts, olives

2. Reduce the amount of the ingredient by half if possible if it cannot be omitted.
   Examples: Shortening, oil, cheese, meat

3. Substitute with a low-fat option.
   Examples: Broth, skim milk, 1% milk, olive oil, canola oil, Butter Buds, Molly McButter, buttermilk, cottage cheese, yogurt, light sour cream, fat-free sour cream

Low Fat Substitutions

Ingredient	Calories	Grams of Fat
Mayonnaise (1 T)	99	11
Nonfat yogurt	8	0
Ground beef (4 oz.)	325	24
Ground turkey	150	0.8

Whole egg	(one)	80	5.5
Egg whites	(two)	30	0
Oil	(1 T)	126	14
Fat-free chicken broth		3	0
Whole milk	(1 c.)	150	8
Skim milk		85	0

Meal Planning

You will feel full very quickly, so you should eat between two and four ounces of food and drink up to six times per day, to start out with, and work up consuming a little more food over time.

Add non-fat dry milk powder whenever you can. Your protein goal is 70 grams per day.

Combinations

You will get full fast, so if you could combine some of the foods, you could assure that you would eat from the various food groups

- Pureed fruit with cottage cheese
- Mashed banana with yogurt
- Mashed banana with a low-fat, low-sugar custard
- Pureed turkey in gravy
- Pureed fish in a thin sauce
- Pureed canned fish in a thin tomato sauce
- Mashed potato in a thin gravy
- Mashed potato with blended low-fat cheese
- Mashed potato with low-fat cream cheese

- Pureed vegetables in chicken soup
- Pureed cottage pie
- Pureed shepherd's pie
- Pureed fish pie
- Pureed mild chili con carne
- Refried beans and low-fat cheese
- Pureed low-fat cottage cheese, vanilla extract, cinnamon, artificial sweetener (for the taste of a cinnamon roll with cream cheese frosting)
- Pureed low-fat cottage cheese (16 ounces) and sugar-free Jell-O powder (1 small envelope)

Alternatively, you could eat things more or less from one food group at a time.

Below is a sample eating schedule that has some things blended together and some food items by themselves:

Menu Idea #1

Breakfast: Sugar-free   Carnation   Instant   Breakfast Essentials, made with skim   milk (6-8 ounces)

Snack: Cottage cheese (.5 cup)

Lunch: Fat-free refried beans (.33 cup) and fat-free/reduced fat cheese (1 ounce, melted) – blended together

Snack: Light yogurt, (4 ounces, blended)

Supper: Meat (.25 cup, if you can tolerate it) and cream soup (.25 cup) and   nonfat   skim   milk powder – blended together

Snack: Skim milk (1 cup) with non-fat dry milk powder (2 tablespoons)

One good method is to have one source of protein and one source of starch at breakfast, one source of protein and one source of fruit at lunch, and one source of protein and one source of vegetables at dinner.

The first menu idea below demonstrates that approach. You may have to eat the second item of each meal as a snack a little later so as to spread out your eating over several tiny meals.

Menu Idea #2

Breakfast:	Protein:	.25 cup pureed scrambled eggs
	Starch:	.25 cup Cream of Wheat
Lunch:	Protein:	.25 cup mashed low fat cottage cheese
	Fruit:	.25 cup pureed peaches
Dinner:	Protein:	.25 cup baked and pureed chicken breast (if tolerated)
	Vegetables:	.25 cup pureed carrots

Menu Idea #3

Breakfast:	Oatmeal with skim milk
Lunch:	Blended chicken (if tolerated) mixed with light mayo
Dinner:	Baked and mashed salmon
Snack:	Mashed peaches with fat-free cottage cheese

Menu Idea #4

Breakfast:	Scrambled and blended eggs
Lunch:	Baked and mashed black beans with fat-free sour cream and mashed avocado
Dinner:	Canned tuna, mashed, with light mayo
Snack:	Low-fat yogurt

Menu Idea #5

Breakfast: Malt O Meal with skim milk

Lunch: Baked and mashed sweet potato

Dinner: Baked and mashed fish

Snack: Shredded and blended low-fat cheese and
              scrambled eggs

Chapter 4:
Ready-Made High Protein, Low Carb, Low Sugar Smoothies and Shakes

You can enjoy many protein smoothies and shakes during this stage.

Of course, it would be better if all of your shakes are created from scratch, but if you want to make things easier for yourself sometimes, there are a few ready-made high protein shakes that are healthy enough for consumption by bariatric patients.

Many protein shake companies advertise the high protein content of their products, but their labels will reveal that they have added a lot of sugar to them. Whether or not that is done to addict the consumer who never ends up losing weight, those drinks are not an option for you.

But for the gastric sleeve patient there are a few good commercially-made protein shake options available that deliver. They are as follows:

1. **MET-Rx Protein Plus** – This company puts out one of the best choices where health benefits are concerned. Their drinks contain 51 grams of protein and only two grams of sugar and 260 calories per drink. Flavor selections include Cookies and Cream, Berry Blast, Mocha Blast, Frosty Chocolate, Peanut Butter, and Creamy Vanilla.

2. **Nature's Best Zero Carb Isopure** – This company's drinks serve up 40 grams of protein and no carbs in just 160 calories. Reports are that the drinks taste good too.

Flavors include Mango Punch, Alpine Punch, Blue Raspberry, Apple Melon, Grape Frost, Icy Orange, Pineapple Orange Banana, and Coconut.

3. **CytoSport Monster Milk** – This drink contains 45 grams of protein, **no sugar** and five grams of dietary fiber. Flavor choices include Vanilla Crème, Cookies and Crème, Chocolate Mint, Chocolate, and Banana Crème.

4. **Muscle Milk Pro** – This one is a favorite one for many bariatric patients because it is easy to obtain. Even some gas stations and convenience stores carry it. The Muscle Milk Pro shakes contain 40 grams of lean protein and two grams of sugar. They are also lactose and gluten free. Flavors include, Mint Chocolate Overload, Knock-Out Chocolate, and Intense Vanilla.

5. **Shakeology** – This drink has many benefits, but the sugar content in it is higher than the sugar included in the other options. These drinks contain 17 grams of protein and six grams of sugar. Added to the benefits of this option are 70 vitamins, minerals, phytonutrients, antioxidants, probiotics, prebiotics, digestive enzymes, and fiber. Flavor selections include Tropical Strawberry Vegan, Strawberry, Greenberry, Vanilla, Vegan Chocolate, and Chocolate.

6. **Pure Protein Shakes** – These drinks contain only 120 calories each but deliver the features that you need in a protein drink. Depending on the size and flavor that you choose, you will get between 23 and 35 grams of protein, one gram of sugar and no aspartame, three grams of fiber, calcium and other benefits. Flavors are limited to just Frosty Chocolate and Vanilla Cream.

Chapter 5:
Smoothie and Shake Recipes for Stage Two of Your Diet

People just love smoothies and shakes. They taste good, satisfy the sweet tooth in us, and they are healthy (if made with the right ingredients). They are also easy to make and convenient.

Most of these recipes call for items with little or no sugar, but some of them do call for fruit, which contains fructose. Peanut butter is often laced with sugar. Try to buy peanut butter that does not have a high amount of sugar in it. Also, you'll want creamy peanut butter instead of crunch because your stomach won't be ready for crunchy nuts.

Be mindful of all of these things when you make your meal replacement drink choices for the week or month and make out your shopping list. You want to concentrate on taking in a high amount of protein and a very low amount of sugar, and you want everything to be soft in consistency.

For any recipe that calls for other nuts, you need to soak the nuts in warm water and then blend them into a cream before you add the other ingredients. Do this while you are recovering from your sugary and then you can just throw the nuts in chopped later on. If they don't taste right creamed and blended into the recipe, simply leave them out!

Don't be afraid to alter recipes or create your own recipes. For instance, maybe you would enjoy creamed cashews better than creamed pecans. Maybe you want to add some greens that are wild edibles, just for added health benefits. Have fun with these recipes. Enjoy their good taste, health, simplicity and convenience. You will likely get hooked on making healthy smoothies and shakes!

When you make your smoothies in your blender, you will need to cut the food into small pieces, use spices and seasonings for flavor, and strain out the lumps and seeds.

Since you won't be consuming much of it during any one meal at first, you may want to blend all ingredients except for the ice, divide the mixture in proportion to the number of ice cubes that the recipe requires, and freeze it until you are about ready to drink it.

When you want a smoothie, take one part of the mixture and one ice cube out and blend them! That way your smoothies will always have the right consistency while also being somewhat premade.

You could use the ice tray idea (Chapter 2) with this most conveniently for measuring in two-ounce segments if you prefer.

Sometimes you won't be hungry, so these high-protein smoothies and shakes are useful because they serve up a lot of protein per ounce because of the protein powder in them.

Kahlua and Scream! Non-Alcoholic Protein Shake

What to Use
- Lactose-free milk (8 ounces)
- Vanilla protein powder (1 scoop)
- Sugar-free DaVinci Kahlua syrup (2-3 pumps/2 tablespoons)
- Sugar-free DaVinci Butter Rum syrup (1-2 pumps/1 tablespoon)
- Ice (3-5 cubes)
- Sugar-free French vanilla pudding mix (optional for creamier consistency)
- Fat-free or sugar-free whipped topping (optional to top off with)

What to Do
- Blend all but the whipped topping and ice for two minutes.
- Then blend in ice, one cube at a time until you like the consistency.
- Pour into glass.
- Top with whipped topping (and umbrella if you have one and are at a party!)

Mexican Chocolate

What to Use
- Cinnamon (.5 teaspoon)
- Almond extract (.5 teaspoon)
- Water or milk (.5 cup)
- Chocolate protein powder (1 scoop)
- Ice cubes (1 cup)

What to Do
- Blend all except ice.
- Add ice and blend.

Cancun Sunset

What to Use
- Frozen strawberries (3 berries)
- Frozen pineapple (1 cube)
- Water or milk (.5 cup)
- Vanilla protein powder (1 scoop)
- Ice cubes (1 cup)

What to Do
- Blend all except ice.
- Add ice and blend.

Peach Cobbler

What to Use
- Ice (4-5 cubes)
- Almond milk (.5 cup, unsweetened)
- Cinnamon (dash)
- Sliced peaches (.5 cup, fresh or frozen)
- Vanilla protein powder (1 scoop)

What to Do
- Blend all except ice.
- Add ice and blend.

Chocolate Covered Cherry

What to Use
- Nutmeg (dash)
- Almond extract (.5 teaspoon)
- Cherries (5 frozen)
- Water or milk (.5 cup)
- Chocolate protein powder (1 scoop)
- Ice cubes (1 cup)

What to Do
- Blend all except ice.
- Add ice and blend.

Chocolate-Peanut Butter-Banana Smoothie

What to Use
- Ice (4-5 cubes)
- Almond milk (.5 cup, unsweetened)
- Vanilla extract (2 teaspoons)
- PB2 (1 tablespoon, regular or chocolate)
- Banana (.5 of banana, frozen)
- Chocolate protein powder (1 scoop)

What to Do
- Blend all except ice.
- Add ice and blend.

Tropical Fruit Protein Smoothie

What to Use
- Ice (4-5 cubes)
- Almond milk (.5 cup, unsweetened)
- Vanilla extract (2 teaspoons)
- Pineapple chunks (2, 1 in cubes)
- Mango chunks (2, 1 in cubes)
- Banana slices (2, 1 in slices)
- Vanilla protein powder (1 scoop)

What to Do
- Blend all except ice.
- Add ice and blend.

Pumpkin Pie Protein Shake

What to Use
- Almond milk (.5 cup, unsweetened)
- Banana (.33 of a banana, frozen)
- Pumpkin pie spice (to taste)
- Pumpkin puree (.25 cup)
- Vanilla protein powder (1 scoop)

Warm Apple Pie Smoothie

What to Use
- Allspice (pinch)
- Nutmeg (pinch)
- Cinnamon (.25 teaspoon)
- Vanilla extract (.25 teaspoon)
- Water (.5 cup)
- Apple (.5 an apple, peeled and cut into cubes)
- Vanilla protein (1 scoop)

What to Do
- Blend all ingredients
- Pour into a mug
- Microwave on high two minutes
- Sprinkle more cinnamon on top

Chunky Monkey

What to Use
- Banana (1, frozen)
- Water or milk (.5 cup)
- Chocolate protein powder (1 scoop)
- Ice cubes (1 cup)

What to Do
- Blend all except ice.
- Add ice and blend.

Cookies and Cream

What to Use
- Vanilla extract (.5 teaspoon)
- Cool whip (1 tablespoon, sugar-free)
- Skim milk (.5 cup)
- Cookies and cream protein (1 scoop)
- Ice cubes (1 cup)

What to Do
- Blend all except ice.
- Add ice and blend.

Cookies and Cream

What to Use
- Vanilla extract (.5 teaspoon)
- Cool Whip (1 tablespoon, sugar-free)
- Skim milk (.5 cup)
- Cookies and cream protein (1 scoop)
- Ice cubes (1 cup)

What to Do
- Blend all except ice.
- Add ice and blend.

Peanut Butter Cup

What to Use
- Peanut butter (2 teaspoons, natural)
- Water or milk (.5 cup)
- Chocolate protein powder (1 cup)
- Ice cubes (1 cup)

What to Do
- Blend all except ice.
- Add ice and blend.

Frozen Latte

What to Use
- Cinnamon (.25 teaspoon)
- Vanilla (.5 teaspoon)
- Water (.5 cup)
- Cappuccino protein (1 cup)
- Ice cubes (1 cup)

What to Do
- Blend all except ice.
- Add ice and blend.

Angel Food Cake Smoothie

What to Use
- Ice (5-6 cubes)
- Almond milk (1 cup, unsweetened)
- Vanilla extract (.5 teaspoon)
- Coconut extract (.5 teaspoon)
- Vanilla protein powder (1 scoop)

What to Do
- Blend all except ice.
- Add ice and blend.

Thin Mint Protein

What to Use
- Peppermint extract (to taste)
- Baby spinach (handful)
- Almond milk (1-1.5 cups, unsweetened)
- Cocoa powder (1 teaspoon)
- Juice chocolate or vanilla protein powder (1 scoop)

Carrot Cake Protein Shake

What to Use
- Almond milk (.5 cup, to taste)
- Banana (.33 of a banana, frozen)
- Carrots (.25 of a carrot, pureed)
- Vanilla protein powder (1 scoop)
- Nutmeg (to taste)
- Ginger (to taste)
- Cinnamon (to taste)

What to Do
- Blend and enjoy!

Lean Mean Green Monster Protein Shake

What to Use
- Banana (.33 of banana, frozen)
- Spinach (3 handfuls, fresh)
- PB2 or peanut butter (2 tablespoons)
- Coffee (.5 cup cold)
- Almond milk (1 cup, unsweetened)
- Vanilla protein powder (1 scoop)

What to Do
- Blend and enjoy!

Pumpkin Protein Shake

What to Use
- Ice cubes (1 cup)
- Cool Whip (.25 cup, sugar-free)
- Splenda Granular (2 tablespoons)
- Pumpkin spice (.25 teaspoon), or cinnamon (.25 teaspoon), or cloves (.125 teaspoon), or ginger (.125 teaspoon)
- Vanilla protein powder (1 scoop, suggestion: Matrix Simply Vanilla)
- Pumpkin puree (.25 cup)
- Skim milk or soy milk (1 cup)

What to Do
- Blend all except ice.
- Add ice and blend.

Mocha Liqueur Shake

What to Use
- Ice (4 cubes)
- Vanilla ice cream (1 pint, sugar-free)
- Protein powder (1 scoop Matrix Simply Vanilla)
- Coffee-flavored liqueur (.25 cup)
- Light rum (.75 cup)

What to Do
- Blend all except ice.
- Add ice and blend.

Maui Martini

Protein: 20 grams

What to Use
- Ice cubes (a few, to taste)
- Banana liqueur (one 1.5-ounce jigger)
- Coconut flavored rum (two 1.5 ounce jiggers)
- Vodka (one 1.5-ounce jigger)
- Vanilla whey protein powder (1 scoop)
- Pineapple for garnish (1 spear or ring, fresh)

What to Do
- Blend all except ice.
- Add ice and blend.

Banana Protein Nog

What to Use
- Vanilla (.5 teaspoon)
- Nutmeg (.125 teaspoon)
- Banana (1-inch chunk)
- Skim milk (1 cup)
- Vanilla protein powder (1 scoop, Matrix Simply Vanilla)

What to Do
- Blend and enjoy!

Banana-Peanut Butter Shake

Protein: 12 grams

What to Use
- Banana (.25 - .5 of a banana)
- Peanut butter (1 tablespoon, creamy)
- Fat-free milk (8 ounces)

What to Do
- Blend and enjoy!

Orange Dreamsicle

Protein: 28 grams

What to Use
- Skim milk (8 ounces; could substitute 4 ounces orange juice or yogurt for 4 ounces of the skim milk)
- Sunrise Orange Crystal Lighta powder (1 scoop/individual serving, sugar-free)
- Vanilla whey protein powder (1 scoop, 20 grams protein)
- Orange zest (.5 teaspoon, optional)

What to Do
- Blend and enjoy!

Sunrise Smoothie

What to Use
- Strawberries (4-5, frozen)
- Splenda (1 tablespoon)
- Low Carb Vanilla Yogurt (1 carton)
- Banana (.5 of a banana)
- Orange juice or orange Tang (1 cup)
- Vanilla protein powder (1 scoop)

What to Do
- Blend and enjoy!

Cherry Vanilla

What to Use
- Cherry sugar-free Kool-Aid (1 cup)
- Low carb vanilla ice cream (2 scoops)
- Maraschino cherries (4-5 cherries)
- Vanilla protein powder (1 scoop)

What to Do
- Blend and enjoy!

Peach

What to Use
- Ice (4 cubes)
- Peach (4-6 slices, fresh)
- Crystal Lite peach tea (1 cup)
- Vanilla protein powder (1 scoop)

What to Do
- Blend all except ice.
- Add ice and blend.

Strawberry-Lemonade

What to Use
- Ice (4-5 cubes)
- Strawberries (4-5 berries, frozen)
- Sugar-free lemonade Kool-Aid (1 cup)
- Vanilla protein powder (1 scoop)

What to Do
- Blend all except ice.
- Add ice and blend.

Cherry Vanilla Coke Float

What to Use
- Cherries (4-5 cherries)
- Diet Coke (1 cup)
- Low-carb sugar-free ice cream (2 scoops)
- Vanilla protein powder (1 scoop)

What to Do
- Blend and enjoy!

Apple Pie Frosty

What to Use
- Ice (8-10 cubes)
- Water (.75 cup)
- Nutmeg (.25 teaspoon)
- Cinnamon (.5 teaspoon)
- Splenda (2 packets)
- Apple (1 apple, peeled, cored, sliced OR .5 cup sugar-free applesauce)
- HDT 5+1 vanilla protein powder (1.5 scoops)

What to Do
- Blend all except ice.
- Add ice and blend.

Butterscotch Pecan Liquid Pie

Calories: 300

What to Use
- Pecans (.25 cups)
- Ice (4-5 cubes)
- Sugar-free butterscotch pudding mix (2 tablespoons)
- Water (8 ounces, cold)
- ProScore 100 vanilla (2 scoops)

What to Do
- Soak pecans in warm water a few hours
- Blend soaked pecans until creamed.
- Blend water, pudding mix and protein powder.
- Add ice. Blend until slivered.
- Pour into parfait glass.

Note: You can just chop the nuts and add last after you get off of your liquid and soft food phase of your post-surgery diet.

Cherry Vanilla Protein Shake

What to Use
- Cherry extract (to taste)
- Vanilla extract (to taste)
- Water (a splash)
- Ice (4 cubes)
- Sugar-free cherry yogurt (.5 cup)
- Vanilla powder (1 scoop)

What to Do
- Blend all except ice.
- Add ice and blend.

Choco Mint Shake

What to Use
- Ice (6 large cubes)
- Water (.5 cup)
- Soy milk (.5 cup)
- Mint flavoring (1 teaspoon)
- Sugar-free hot chocolate mix (1 packet)
- HDT 5+1 chocolate protein powder (1.5 scoops)

What to Do
- Blend all except ice.
- Add ice and blend.

Chocolate Almond Shake

What to Use
- Ice (6-8 cubes)
- Almonds (.25 cup)
- Almond flavoring (1 teaspoon)
- Sweet and Low chocolate syrup (2 tablespoons)
- Soy milk (1 cup)
- ProScore 100 chocolate (2 scoops)

What to Do
- Soak almonds in warm water a few hours.
- Cream almonds in blender.
- Add and blend everything else except for the ice.
- Add ice and blend.

Chocolate Banana Peanut Butter De-Lite

What to Use
- Sugar-free white chocolate instant pudding mix (1 tablespoon)
- Low-sugar peanut butter (1 tablespoon)
- Banana (.5 of a small banana)
- PS IOO chocolate protein powder (2 scoops)
- Equal (4 packets)
- Toasted marshmallow sugar-free syrup (.25 cup)
- Water (.75 cup, cold)

What to Do
- Blend and enjoy!

Chocolate Banana Smoothie

What to Use
- Chocolate protein powder (1 scoop)
- Vanilla extract (dash)
- Banana (.5 cup, sliced, ripe)
- Non-fat milk (.5 cup)
- Banana fat-free NutraSweet-sweetened yogurt (.5 cup)

What to Do
- Blend and enjoy!

Chocolate Coconut Shake

What to Use
- Chocolate or banana sugar-free pudding (1 teaspoon)
- Chocolate protein powder (2 scoops)
- Water (6 ounces, cold)
- Coconut milk (2 ounces)

What to Do
- Hand shake well.

Chocolate Covered Banana

What to Use
- Ice (2 handfuls)
- Maraschino cherries (4 cherries)
- Banana (.5 of a banana)
- Sugar-free chocolate syrup (splash)
- 1% milk (.5 cup)
- Chocolate Isopure (1 scoop)

What to Do
- Blend all except ice.
- Add ice and blend.

Chocolate Covered Cherry Shake

What to Use
- Ice (8-10 cubes)
- Cherries (10-12 cherries, no pits)
- Sweet N Low chocolate syrup (2 tablespoons)
- Soy milk (1 cup)
- HDT 5+1 chocolate protein powder (1.5 scoops)

What to Do
- Blend all except ice.
- Add ice and blend.

Chocolate Frosty Shake

What to Use
- Ice (10 cubes)
- Fat-free non-dairy coffee creamer (1 rounded teaspoon, powder)
- Fat-free sugar-free French Vanilla International Coffee (1 rounded teaspoon)
- Chocolate protein powder (1 rounded scoop)

What to Do
- Blend all except ice.
- Add ice and blend.

Chocolate Fudge Shake

What to Use
- Ice (5 large cubes)
- Water (8 ounces)
- Chocolate fudge sugar-free pudding mix (2 tablespoons)
- ProScore 100 chocolate (2 scoops)

What to Do
- Blend together all but the ice.
- Add ice and blend until slivered

Chocolate OrangeSicle

What to Use
- Water (8 ounces)
- OrangeSicle protein powder (.5 scoop)
- ProScore 100 chocolate (1.5 scoops)

What to Do
- Blend and enjoy!

Chocolate Peanut Butter Death

What to Use
- Ice (6 ounces, crushed)
- Peanut butter (1 heaping tablespoon, reduced fat creamy)
- Fat-free Cool Whip Light (1 heaping tablespoon)
- Sugar-free DaVinci Cookie Dough Syrup (1.5 ounces)
- Sugar-free DaVinci Peanut Butter Syrup (1.5 ounces)
- Splenda (1 packet)
- Chocolate sugar-free pudding mix (2 teaspoons)
- PS100 Chocolate Protein Powder (2 scoops)
- Water (8 ounces, cold)

What to Do
- Blend all except ice.
- Add ice and blend.

Chocolate Peanut Butter Shake

What to Use
- Chocolate protein powder (1 scoop)
- Peanut butter (1 tablespoon, creamy)
- Skim milk (1 cup)
- Ice (2 handfuls)

What to Do
- Blend all except ice.
- Add ice and blend.

Chocolate Raspberry Shake

What to Use
- ProScore 100 chocolate (2 scoops)
- Water or skim, lactaid or soy milk (8 ounces)
- Sugar-free raspberry syrup (to taste)

What to Do
- Blend and enjoy!

Chocolate Vanilla Swirl

What to Use
- Chocolate protein powder (.5 scoop)
- Vanilla protein powder (.5 scoop)
- Vitamite (splash)
- Water (splash)
- Ice (to taste)

What to Do
- Blend all except ice.
- Add ice and blend.

Chocolate-Banana Shake

What to Use
- Ice (2 handfuls)
- Skim milk (1 cup)
- Banana (.5 of a banana)
- Chocolate protein powder (1 scoop)

What to Do
- Blend all except ice.
- Add ice and blend.

Coco Loco

What to Use
- Ice (5 cubes)
- Rum extract (1 drop, optional)
- Pineapple extract (2 drops)
- Coconut extract (2 drops)
- Luzianne Peach Mango ice tea flavoring (splash)
- Splenda (6 packets)
- Vitamite (4 ounces)
- 100% Whey Vanilla Protein powder (1.5 scoops)

What to Do
- Blend all except ice.
- Add ice and blend.

Cookies and Cream

What to Use
- ProBlend 55 (.33 scoop)
- Sugar-free DaVinci Chocolate Chip Cookie Dough Syrup (1 teaspoon)
- Water (splash)
- Cookies and Cream coffee (splash)
- Vitamite (splash)

What to Do
- Blend and enjoy!

Mocha/Cappuccino

What to Use
- Pro V60 Vanilla Crème Ice Blend (.33 scoop)
- Pro V60 Chocolate Thunder (.33 scoop)

What to Do
- Blend and enjoy!

Creamy Peach Melba

What to Use
- Keto Peaches and Cream Protein Powder (2 scoops)
- Heavy cream (1 tablespoon)
- Splenda (2 packets)
- DaVinci raspberry flavor (1 teaspoon)
- Peach mango Luzianne tea flavor (1 tablespoon)
- Water (4-6 ounces)
- Peach slices (6-8 slices, frozen)

What to Do
- Blend the peaches, flavorings, Splenda and water.
- Add protein powder.
- Drizzle the cream in last and blend well.

Donna's Delicious Protein Smoothie

What to Use
- Vanilla protein powder (1 scoop)
- Raspberries (1 scoop, frozen)
- Ice (3 cubes)
- Sunrise Orange Crystal Light (6-8 ounces, premade)
- Cool Whip (sugar free, optional)

What to Do
- Blend the Crystal Light, ice and raspberries.
- Add the protein and blend just a few seconds to prevent it from foaming.

Double Chocolate Fudge

What to Use
- Ice (4 cubes or .5-1 cup crushed)
- Chocolate protein powder (1 scoop)
- Sugar-free hot cocoa mix (1 packet)
- Skim milk (.5 cup)

What to Do
- Blend all except ice.
- Add ice and blend.

Egg Nog

What to Use
- Ice (4-6 cubes)
- Allspice (.5 teaspoon)
- Rum extract (1 teaspoon)
- Vanilla HDT 5+1 (1 scoop)
- Soy milk (1 cup)

What to Do
- Blend all except ice.
- Add ice and blend.

Elvis in My Kitchen

What to Use
- Peanut butter (1 tablespoon, creamy)
- Ice (3-5 cubes)
- Raspberry or peach or other sugar-free syrup (1 tablespoon)
- Water (8 ounces)
- Vanilla sugar-free instant pudding (1 tablespoon)
- ProScore Vanilla Protein Powder (2 scoops)

What to Do
- Blend the syrup, protein powder, and pudding.
- Add ice and blend until slivered.
- Add peanut butter and blend a few seconds.

Extra Spicy ProScore mocha Chai

What to Use
- Vanilla extract (splash)
- Nutmeg (pinch)
- ProScore 100 Chocolate Protein Powder (2 scoops)
- Ice (4-5 cubes)
- Unsweetened Chai tea (1 ounce, cold and strong)
- Peppercorns (4-5 cloves)
- Ginger (1 piece, fresh)
- Coffee with Half & Half (2 ounces, cold and strong)

What to Do
- Blend the coffee, tea, peppercorns, cloves and ginger.
- Blend ice, adding them one at a time, until they are broken up.
- Add protein powder while blender is on.
- Add the vanilla, nutmeg and cinnamon.

Frappaccino

What to Use
- Skim milk (.5 cup)
- Ice (2 handfuls)
- Chocolate or vanilla protein powder (1 scoop)
- Instant coffee or cold coffee (1 tablespoon)

What to Do
- Blend all except ice.
- Add ice and blend.

Frappuccino On-the-Go

What to Use
- Chocolate protein powder (1 scoop)
- Blue Luna Light Mocha (.5 can, can use Starbuck's Light Frappaccino)

What to Do
- Mix and pour over ice.

Fudgesicle

What to Use
- Ice (6 cubes)
- DaVinci sugar-free vanilla syrup (.5 ounce)
- Sugar-free fudgesicle (one)
- Splenda (10 packets)
- Water (12 ounces, cold)
- Chocolate protein powder (1.5 scoops)

What to Do
- Blend on high all ingredients except for the protein.
- Turn speed down, add protein, and replace lid.
- Blend, but not on high.

Good Morning Smoothie

What to Use
- Vanilla protein powder (1 scoop)
- Orange juice (.25 cup, fresh squeezed)
- Non-fat sugar-free strawberry yogurt (.5 cup)
- Skim milk (.75 cup)
- Banana (1 small)

What to Do
- Blend all ingredients except for ice.
- Add ice and blend.

Iced Mocha Latte

What to Use
- Ice (a few cubes)
- Sugar-free hazelnut coffee syrup (splash)
- Fat-free sugar-free vanilla pudding mix (1 tablespoon)
- ProScore 100 chocolate (2 scoops)
- Coffee (to taste, cold; could use decaf Hazelnut)

What to Do
- Blend all except ice.
- Add ice and blend.

Light and Dark Syphony

What to Use
- Water (splash, ice cold)
- Coffee (splash)
- ProBlend 55 Mocha Cappuccino (1 scoop)
- White chocolate sugar-free syrup (1 tablespoon, optional...for dark symphony)

What to Do
- Blend and enjoy!

Luscious Pina Colada

What to Use
- Ice
- Pineapple flavoring (dash)
- Coconut flavoring (dash)
- Vanilla sugar-free pudding mix (2 tablespoon)
- ProScore 100 vanilla (2 scoops)

What to Do
- Blend all except ice.
- Add ice and blend.

Mango Morning Smoothie

What to Use
- ProScore Vanilla (2 scoops)
- Ice (7-8 cubes)
- Vanilla or almond extract (1 teaspoon)
- Ginger (small piece, fresh)
- Mango (1, meat part)
- Water (2 ounces, cold)
- Lime (fresh-squeezed juice from .5 of lime)

What to Do
- Blend everything except protein and ice.
- Add protein while blender is on.
- Add ice one cube at a time.

Mocha, Ginger and Cinnamon

What to Use
- Ginger (small piece, fresh)
- Ice (6-8 cubes)
- Cinnamon (a few sprinkles)
- Coffee with Half and Half (4 ounces cold)
- ProScore 100 Chocolate (2 scoops)

What to Do
- Blend on low. Then blend on high.
- Throw ice in, one cube at a time while blending.

Old Fashioned Vanilla Ice Cream Shake

What to Use
- Ice cubes ("lots")
- Vitamite (5 ounces)
- DaVinci's Sugar-Free Vanilla Syrup (1 capful)
- Splenda (4-5 packets)
- GNC 100% Whey Vanilla Protein Powder (1.5 scoop)

What to Do
- Blend all together except for protein powder and ice.
- Add the protein powder and blend.
- Add ice and blend until well-chopped.

Orange and Cream Shake

What to Use
- ProV60 Vanilla Cream protein (1 scoop)
- Vitamite (splash)
- Stewart's Diet Orange and Cram Soda (8 ounces or less)
- Ice (to taste)

What to Do
- Blend extra thoroughly to take out the carbonation.

Orange Banana Smoothie

What to Use
- Ice (1 cup)
- Keto Shake Banana Crème protein powder (1 rounded scoop)
- Keto Shake Orange Crème protein powder (1 rounded scoop)
- Banana (.5 of a banana, sliced)
- Orange juice (.5 cup, no pulp)
- Water (.5 cup, cold)
- Ice (1 cup)

What to Do
- Blend all except for the ice.
- Add the ice.

Orange Julius

What to Use
- Protein powder (2 scoops)
- Vanilla extract (1 tablespoon)
- Skim milk (2.5 cups)
- Frozen orange juice concentrate (one 6-ounce can)
- Non-fat plain yogurt (8-ounces)

What to Do
- Blend and enjoy!

Orange Julius, Nuthin' on Us Smoothie

What to Use
- Ice (3-4 cubes)
- Vanilla flavoring (1 teaspoon)
- Orange juice (.25 cup fresh squeezed with pulp)
- Sugar-free vanilla pudding mix (1 tablespoon)
- Water (6 ounces)
- ProScore 100 vanilla (2 scoops)

What to Do
- Blend all except for the ice.
- Add ice. Blend until ice slivers.

Peach Creamsicle

What to Use
- Ice (cubes, to taste)
- Splenda (6 packets)
- Vanilla protein powder (1 scoop)
- Sugar-free instant vanilla pudding (2 tablespoons)
- Crystal Lite Peach Tea (6 ounces)

What to Do
- Blend all except ice.
- Add ice and blend.

Peach and Strawberry Yummy

What to Use
- Vanilla protein powder (1 rounded)
- Splenda (1 packet)
- Water (.25 - .5 cup)
- Strawberries (3 large berries, frozen)
- Peaches (3 slices) or .5 of a banana

What to Do
- Blend and enjoy!

Pina Colada Smoothie

What to Use
- Vanilla protein powder (1 scoop)
- Artificial sweetener (1 packet)
- Ice (.5 cup, crushed)
- Coconut extract (1 tablespoon)
- Crushed pineapple in unsweetened juice (one 8-ounce can, refrigerated)

What to Do
- Blend all except ice.
- Add ice and blend.

Pineapple Vanilla Ginger Shake

What to Use
- ProScore 100 Vanilla Protein Powder
- Ice (5-6 cubes)
- Ginger (1 small piece, fresh)
- Pineapple (.5 small, cold with enough water to blend)
- Cinnamon (to taste)
- Mint (fresh, to taste)
- Ginger (to taste)
- Water (enough to blend)

What to Do
- Blend the pineapple first with a little water and ginger.
- Add ice one cube at a time until creamy.
- Add the protein while blender is on.
- Pour into brandy glass, and sprinkle with the cinnamon and fresh mint.

Real Root Beer Float

What to Use
- Diet Root Beer (.75 of the can)
- Vanilla protein powder (1 scoop)
- Sugar-free vanilla ice cream (1.5 scoops)

What to Do
- Stir thoroughly

Root Beer Float

What to Use
- Diet Root Beer (1 can)
- Vanilla protein powder (1 scoop)

What to Do
- Blend and enjoy!

Enen Better Root Beer Float

What to Use
- Splenda (2 envelopes)
- Ice (4-5 cubes)
- Diet Root Beer (one 12-ounce can, flat (no carbonation left in it)
- Vanilla Carb Solutions Protein Powder (2 scoops)

What to Do
- Blend all except ice.
- Add ice and blend.

S'Mores

What to Use
- ProV60 Chocolate Thunder protein powder
- DaVinci Sugar-Free Toasted Marshmallow Syrup (to taste)
- Vitamite (splash)
- Coffee (to taste, optional)
- Sans Sucre Cinnamon-Sugar (to taste)
- Ice (to taste)

What to Do
- Blend all except ice.
- Add ice and blend.

Snicker

What to Use
- Ice (to taste)
- Chocolate protein powder (1 scoop)
- Vitamite (splash)
- Snicker Doodle Coffee (splash), or sugar-free hazelnut syrup and sugar-   free cinnamon-sugar
- Water (splash)

What to Do
- Blend all except ice.
- Add ice and blend.

Snickers Candy Bar

What to Use
- Ice (to taste)
- Chocolate protein powder (to taste)
- Peanut butter (1 teaspoon), or sugar-free peanut butter syrup
- Water (splash)
- Vitamite (splash)
- Chocolate caramel coffee (splash), or regular coffee, sugar-free caramel syrup, or sugar-free chocolate syrup (for more chocolate taste)

What to Do
- Blend all except ice.
- Add ice and blend.

Strawberry Berry

What to Use
- Ice (1 cup, crushed or cubed)
- Cranberry juice (1 cup)
- Blueberries (.25 cup)
- Strawberries (4 berries, frozen or fresh)
- Strawberry Pro Blend 55 (1 scoop)

What to Do
- Blend all except ice.
- Add ice and blend.

Strawberry Chocolate Milk

What to Use
- Water (14 ounces(
- Carnation Fat-Free Hot Cocoa
- Carb Solutions (1 scoop)
- Strawberry Carb Solutions (2 scoops)

What to Do
- Blend and enjoy!

Strawberry for Protein Dummies

What to Use
- Splenda (to taste)
- Water (8 ounces)
- Biochem's Ultimate LO Carb Whey (1 scoop, natural flavor)
- Banana (.5 of a small banana)
- Strawberries (10 berries, frozen)

What to Do
- Blend and enjoy!

Tropical Breakfast Smoothie

What to Use
- Vanilla protein powder (1 scoop)
- Cholesterol-free egg product (.5 cup)
- Banana (1 banana, sliced, fresh)
- Pineapple chunks in natural juice (8 ounces)
- Strawberries (1 cup, cut up, fresh)

What to Do
- Blend and enjoy!

Two Berry Delight

What to Use
- Orange protein powder or orange juice vitamins (1 cup)
- Milk (.5 cup)
- Sweetener (1 packet)
- Ice (1 cup)
- Raspberries (.5 cup)
- Strawberries (1 cup, frozen or fresh)

What to Do
- Blend all ingredients except for the ice.
- Add ice and blend.

Vanilla Butterscotch

What to Use
- Ice (4-5 cubes)
- Vanilla sugar-free pudding (1 tablespoon)
- Butterscotch sugar-free pudding (1 tablespoon)
- Vanilla ProScore (2 scoops)
- Water (8 ounces, cold)
- Vanilla butterscotch (to taste)

What to Do
- Blend all ingredients except for the ice.
- Add the ice and blend.
- Let it set up a little. It tastes like custard.

Vanilla Chai

What to Use
- Soy milk (splash)
- Splenda (a little)
- Cinnamon (dash)
- Chai tea (8 ounces, made from a tea bag, refrigerated)
- Vanilla protein powder

What to Do
- Blend and enjoy!

Vanilla Frosty

What to Use
- Ice (10-12 cubes)
- Water or soy milk (.75 cup)
- Dannon Fit and Light Yogurt (.5 – 1 container, any flavor)
- HDT 5+1 vanilla protein powder (1.5 scoops)

What to Do
- Blend all except ice.
- Add ice and blend.

Vanilla PB Fruity

What to Use
- Ice (3-5 cubes)
- Peanut butter (2 teaspoons)
- Sugar-free syrup, any flavor (1 tablespoon)
- Water (8 ounces)
- Sugar-free vanilla pudding mix (1 tablespoon)
- ProScore 100 vanilla (2 scoops)

What to Do
- Blend all ingredients except for the ice and peanut butter.
- Add ice and blend until the ice slivers.
- Add the peanut butter and blend briefly.

Vanilla Spice Freeze

What to Use
- Cloves (pinch)
- Cinnamon (pinch)
- Vanilla sugar-free pudding mix (2 tablespoons)
- ProScore 100 vanilla (2 scoops)

What to Do
- Blend. Put into freezer until thick. Then eat.

Vanilla Citrus

What to Use
- ProScore 100 Vanilla (2 scoops)
- Ice (6 cubes)
- Vanilla extract (.5 teaspoon)
- Ginger (to taste, fresh)
- Lime (.25 of lime including rind, cut into 5 pieces
- Water (2 ounces, cold)
- Cinnamon (to taste)

What to Do
- Blend all except ice.
- Add ice and blend.

White Chocolate Mouse Mocha Frappaccino

What to Use
- Ice (handful)
- Sugar-free Jell-O White Chocolate Mouse Pudding (.5 teaspoon)
- PB55 Mocha Frappachino
- Water (splash)
- Vitamite (splash)

What to Do
- Blend all except ice.
- Add ice and blend.

Vanilla Protein "Milkshake"

What to Use
- Ice (5-10 cubes, depending on desired thickness)
- Sweetener (to taste)
- Low-fat cottage cheese (.5 cup)
- Unsweetened vanilla almond milk (.5 cup)
- Vanilla protein powder (1 scoop)
- Vanilla extract (.25 teaspoon)
- Flavor options: strawberries (.25 cup, frozen); banana (.5 a banana); cocoa powder (2 tablespoons); sugar-free pudding mix (2-3 tablespoons)

What to Do
- Blend all except ice.
- Add ice and blend.

Apple Pie Protein Shake

What to Use
- Ice (4-6 cubes)
- Cinnamon (dash)
- Vanilla protein powder (1 scoop)
- Water (1 cup)
- Apple cider mix (1 packet)

What to Do
- Blend all except ice.
- Add ice and blend.

Spicy Autumn Smoothie

What to Use
- WonderSlim Vanilla Cream Puddin/Shake Mix (1 packet)
- Artificial sweetener (to taste)
- Cinnamon (.125 teaspoon)
- Nutmeg (.125 teaspoon)
- Banana (.5 cup)
- Yams (.5 cup)
- Water (1 cup)
- Ice (2-6 cubes)

What to Do
- Blend all except ice.
- Add ice and blend.

Peanut Butter and Jelly Protein Smoothie

What to Use
- Berries (1 cup, frozen)
- Natural peanut butter (1 tablespoon)
- Vanilla Bean, Designer Whey Sustained Energy (1 scoop)
- Rolled oats (2 tablespoons)
- Soy milk (1 cup)

What to Do
- Blend until smooth.

Spinach Flax Protein Smoothie

What to Use
- Vanilla protein powder (optional)
- Chia seeds (optional)
- Flax meal (optional)
- Banana (.5 of a banana, fresh or frozen)
- Pineapple (.25 cup, frozen)
- Mango (.25 cup, frozen chunks)
- Baby spinach (1 large handful, organic, washed)
- Almond milk (1 cup, unsweetened)

What to Do
- Alter ingredient amounts to suit your taste
- Blend until smooth
- Serve immediately

Dark Chocolate Peppermint Protein Shake

What to Use
- Designer Whey Gourmet Chocolate Protein Powder (1 scoop)
- Non-dairy milk (1 cup, milk of choice)
- Banana (1 large, frozen)
- Cocoa powder (2 tablespoons)
- Sea salt (pinch)
- Pure peppermint extract (.25 teaspoon)
- Vegan whipped cream or Greek yogurt (to taste, as a topping)
- Ice (2-3 large cubes)

What to Do
- Blend together until smooth

Almond Butter Chia Smoothie

What to Use
- Almond butter (1 tablespoon)
- Unsweetened almond milk (1 tablespoon)
- Banana (1 large ripe banana, peeled and frozen)
- Chia seeds (1 tablespoon, ASK YOUR DOCTOR)
- Cinnamon (to taste, ground, optional)
- Maca powder (to taste, optional)
- Raw cacao powder (to taste, optional)
- Blueberries (to taste, optional)
- Spinach (to taste, optional)

What to Do
- Blend all together until smooth

Blueberry and Grape Protein Smoothie

What to Use
- Banana (1 ripe, peeled and frozen)
- Egg (1 beaten, scrambled and frozen)
- Blueberries (.5 cup, fresh)
- Red grapes (.5 cup, frozen)
- Almond milk (1 cup, unsweetened)
- Orange juice (.25 cup)
- Cinnamon (.125 - .25 teaspoon, ground)
- Ice (3 large cubes)

What to Do
- Scramble the egg over medium heat. Cool
- Blend all ingredients together.

French Toast Protein Shake

What to Use
- Fat-free cottage cheese (.5 cup)
- Vanilla protein powder (1 scoop)
- Sugar-free maple extract (2 tablespoons)
- Cinnamon (.5 teaspoon)
- Pumpkin pie spice or nutmeg (dash)
- Stevia (3-5 packets)
- Water (.5 – 1 cup, to desired consistency)
- Xanthan gum (.5 teaspoon)
- Butter extract (.5 teaspoon)
- Ice (5-10 cubes, to desired thickness)

What to Do
- Blend
- Top with sugar-free whipped topping and cinnamon, if desired

Chocolate Banana Peanut Butter Breakfast Shake

What to Use
- Bananas (2 large overripe, but not black, bananas, peeled, sliced and frozen)
- Almond milk (1 cup original)
- Peanut butter (.25 cup, creamy)
- Unsweetened cocoa powder (2 tablespoons)
- Vanilla extract (.5 teaspoons)
- Ice (.75 cup)

What to Do
- Blend all ingredients
- Serve immediately

Blueberry-Almond Butter Smoothie

What to Use
- Banana (1 banana, peeled)
- Bluberries (1 cup, frozen)
- Almond butter (.5 cup)
- Plain yogurt (.5 cup)
- Almond milk (.75 cup)
- Dates (3, pitted and quartered)
- Ice (1 cup or as needed)

What to Do
- Blend all ingredients except for ice.
- Add ice a cube at a time until the desired consistency is reached.

Raw Banana Bread Shake

What to Use

- Walnut milk (3 cups)
- Banana (2 cups, sliced, fresh or frozen)
- Cinnamon (1 teaspoon, ground)
- Nutmeg (pinch, grated, fresh)
- Vanilla extract (.5 teaspoon)
- Ice (optional)

What to Do

- Soak walnuts a few hours.
- Put walnuts into blender and blend until creamy.
- Add enough filtered water to make three cups.
- Strain the walnut "milk" with a fine mesh strainer and keep the milk in the refrigerator until you are ready to use it. It separates, so shake when you take it out to use it.
- Blend all ingredients together when ready to make a shake.

Peach and Oat Breakfast Smoothie

What to Use

- Peaches (1.5 cups, peeled and diced, frozen)
- Almond and coconut milk blend, or original almond milk (1 cup)
- Greek yogurt (5.3 ounce; mango, peach, strawberry or coconut)
- Banana (1 very ripe banana, peeled and frozen)
- Oats (.5 cup, old fashioned or quick)
- Water (.5 cup, cold)

What to Do

- Blend all ingredients until well-pureed.
- Serve immediately.

Orange Julius Protein Smoothie

What to Use
- Low-fat cottage cheese or Greek yogurt (1 cup)
- Orange zest (zest of one orange)
- Orange juice (4 tablespoons)
- Strawberries (1 cup, frozen)
- Stevia (2-3 packets)
- Almond milk (1 cup, unsweetened)
- Ice (.5 – 1 cup cubes)

What to Do
- Note: You could 2 scoops of protein powder and 2 frozen bananas or else coconut yogurt in place of almond milk, if desired.
- Blend all ingredients until smooth.

Fresh Blueberry Smoothie

What to Use
- Almond milk (.5 cup, unsweetened)
- Vanilla plant-based protein powder (1 scoop)
- Blueberries (.5 cup, frozen)
- Almond butter (.5 tablespoon natural, unsalted)
- Water (optional, to blend)

What to Do
- Blend until smooth.

Peanut Butter Cup

What to Use
- Almond milk (.5 cup, unsweetened)
- Vanilla or chocolate protein powder (1 scoop, plant-based)
- Cocoa powder (1 tablespoon, unsweetened)
- Banana (.5 a banana, frozen)
- Peanut butter (.5 tablespoon, natural and unsalted)
- Water (optional, to blend)

What to Do
- Blend until creamy

Green Monster

What to Use
- Apple juice (.25 cup, no sugar added)
- Water (.25 cup)
- Vanilla protein powder (.5 scoop, plant-based)
- Bosc pear (.5 pear chopped)
- Baby spinach (.5 cup, loosely packed)
- Banana (.5 banana, frozen)
- Avocado (.25 avocado, ripe)

What to Do
- Blend all ingredients until smooth.

Dreamy Creamsicle

What to Use
- Diet orange soda (8 ounces, flat)
- Vanilla protein powder (1 scoop)
- Vanilla yogurt cubes (4 frozen low-fat)

What to Do
- Blend until smooth.

Chapter 6:
Blended Meat Meal Recipes for Stage Two of Your Diet Following Gastric Sleeve Surgery

Pureed Meal Recipes

You may or may not tolerate meat at first. Still, you may be hungry for a meal that contains meat and want some normal-tasting meals once in a while. Some of these kinds of meals can call for too many carbs. Feel free to alter the recipes so as to not eat too many carbs.

Avocado, Chicken and Potato

Protein: 9 grams
Carbohydrate: 14 grams
Calories: 130

What to Use
- Skim milk (2 teaspoons)
- Avocado (.5 of avocado, ripe)
- Chicken (50 g / 2 ounces, boneless thigh or breast)
- Potato (300 g / 11 ounces before peeled, peeled and cut into chunks)
- Salt (to taste)

- Pepper (to taste, freshly ground)

What to Do
- Steam chicken and potato together 25-30 minutes, or cook in microwave.
- Blend the chicken, potato and all of the other ingredients together.
- Thin with milk if runnier consistency is needed.

Maryland Shrimp Spread

Protein: 15 grams
Net carbs: 4 grams
Fats: 3 grams
Calories: 73

What to Use
- Old Bay Seasoning (1 teaspoon)
- Scallions (3, chopped)
- Hellmann's Reduced Fat mayo (.25 cup)
- Shrimp (1 pound, cooked)

What to Do
- Blend shrimp, leaving slightly chunky. Transfer to bowl.
- Blend scallions, mayo and Old Bay together.
- Mix all together, adding water to make into the consistency of applesauce while you are in stage two of your post-surgery diet.

Pinto Bean Dip

Protein: 9 grams
Net carbs: 10 grams
Fats: 3 grams
Calories: 65 grams

What to Use
- Chicken broth (.5 cup)
- Salsa (1 cup)
- Pinto beans (1 15-ounce can, drained and rinsed)
- Olive oil (2 teaspoons)
- Garlic (2 cloves, chopped)
- Onion (1 small, diced)

What to Do
- Saute garlic and onion in the olive oil until golden brown.
- Blend the beans, sautéed veggies and the salsa.
- Add broth a little at a time until you reach the consistency of applesauce while you are in stage two of your post-operation diet.
- Cook mixture in skillet about 10 minutes, until bubbly and thickened.

Mashed White Beans with Garlic and Rosemary

Protein: 8 grams
Net carbs: 13 grams
Fats: 5 grams
Calories: 169

What to Use
- Olive oil (3 tablespoons)
- Garlic (2 large cloves, peeled but whole)
- Rosemary (1 sprig, fresh)
- Cannellini beans (two 14-ounce cans, drained and rinsed)
- Chicken broth (1-2 tablespoons)
- Parmesan cheese (1 tablespoons, freshly grated)
- Kosher salt and pepper

What to Do
- Heat up the olive oil to medium heat.
- Saute the garlic and rosemary sprig until the rosemary is crispy and the garlic is soft.
- Mash or blend the garlic.
- Take the rosemary off to the side. Take the leaves off, mince them and return them to the skillet.
- Add the beans and heat them through. Stir and mash or blend the beans.
- Add chicken broth until you reach the consistency of applesauce (while you are in stage two of your post-operation diet).
- Add the Parmesan, salt a pepper. Stir.
- Place into serving bowl. Drizzle with extra olive oil.

Butternut Squash, Black Bean and Kale Quesadillas

What to Use
- Part-skim mozzarella cheese (1.5 cups, shredded)
- Black beans (1 cup canned unsalted, rinsed and drained)
- Salt (.25 teaspoon)
- Canola oil (1 teaspoon)
- Baby kale (2 cups)
- Water (2 cups)
- Butternut squash (2 cups, pre-chopped and peeled

What to Do
- Heat skillet to medium heat.
- Add 6 tablespoons of water and the squash. Cover. Cook for 6 minutes.
- Uncover. Stir in the oil, salt and kale. Cook for 2 minutes.
- Remove from heat.
- Put the beans and the squash mixture in a bowl and mash them.
- Melt the cheese in it and serve.
- Once you are off of your diet, you can put this between whole wheat flour tortillas (four 8-inch)

Thirty-Minute Chicken Curry

What to Use
- Chopped cilantro leaves (.25 cup)
- Coconut creamer or fat-free Half and Half (.5 cup)
- Turmeric (.25 teaspoon)
- Curry (2 teaspoons)
- Peanut butter (2 tablespoons, natural and creamy)
- Coconut milk (one 13.5-ounce can)
- Cornstarch (1 tablespoon)
- Chicken broth (1 cup)
- Chicken (3 cups cooked and blended)
- Garlic (3 cloves, minced)
- Carrots (1 cup, shredded)
- Red bell pepper, (1 medium, diced)
- Sesame oil (1 tablespoon)

What to Do
- Heat sesame oil in a large skillet. Heat to medium high heat.
- Add bell pepper, carrots, garlic and green onion. Cook for 3-4 minutes or until slightly tender.
- Blend the cooked vegetables in your blender. Return to the skillet.
- Add the cooked and blended chicken to the skillet and stir together.
- In a bowl, whisk together the broth and cornstarch. Pour over the veggie and chicken mixture in the skillet. Bring to a boil. Reduce heat to medium-low. Simmer 1-2 minutes.
- Add the peanut butter, milk, turmeric, curry and sriracha. Mix together. Simmer for 5 minutes.
- Stir in coconut creamer and the chopped cilantro just before serving, cooking it for a minute so as to heat it through.
- Once you are off of your post-surgery diet, you can top it with coconut, peanuts and cilantro leaves.

Thirty-Minute Salmon en Papillote

What to Use
- Sea salt
- Black pepper (freshly ground)
- Lemon juice (of .5 a lemon)
- Dill (1 package, fresh)
- Herbes de Provence (.5 teaspoon)
- Wild salmon fillet (1 pound, skin removed)
- Shallot (1, sliced)
- Zucchini (1 medium, sliced)

What to Do
- Preheat oven to 350 degrees Fahrenheit.
- Cut parchment paper to fit your baking sheet.
- Place the shallots and zucchini on half of the paper. Season with sea salt and pepper. Toss and coat evenly with fingers.
- Put salmon on top of the shallots and zucchini. Season salmon with Herbes de Provence, sea salt and pepper. Put dill and squeezed lemon juice on the very top.
- Fold over the parchment paper and seal it well by folding small sections all the way around. You don't want any of the steam to escape.
- Bake 15-20 minutes.
- While you are in stage two of your diet, you can blend the veggies together and then mash or blend the salmon, or you could blend the veggies and the salmon together.

Baked Chicken Meatballs with BBQ Sauce

What to Use

Meatballs:
- Chicken (1 pound, ground lean)
- Red pepper (.25 medium, seeded)
- Carrot (.25 cup, shredded)
- Red onion (.25 medium)
- Eggs (1 large, beaten)
- Breadcrumbs (.75 cup, Italian-seasoned)
- Parsley (.25 cup, Italian flat-leaf)
- Garlic (2 cloves)
- Sea salt (.5 teaspoon)
- Black pepper (.25 teaspoon)

BBQ Sauce:
- Liquid smoke (1 tablespoon)
- Sugar-free brown sugar (2 tablespoons)
- Worcestershire sauce (2 tablespoons)
- Reduced-sodium soy sauce (.25 cup)
- Beef broth (1 cup)
- Sugar-free ketchup (2 cups)

What to Do

- Preheat oven to 400 degree Fahrenheit. Line baking sheet with parchment paper.
- Mix together the chicken, egg and bread crumbs in a bowl. Set it aside.
- Cut open the red pepper and take the seeds out of it. You don't want to eat the seeds.
- Blend the garlic, parsley, red pepper, carrot and red onion in blender until very finely chopped
- Add to the chicken. Mix, but do not overly mix them or they may turn out to be hard.
- Form the chicken and vegetable mixture into meatballs the size of golf balls. Place them on the baking sheet.
- Bake them for 15 minutes or until cooked through.
- While the meatballs are baking, put all ingredients for the BBQ sauce in a large skillet and heat over medium heat.
- When you are off of your diet, you could just roll each meatball in the sauce after the meat balls are baked through and eat them that way. But while you are in the second stage of your post-surgery diet, you'll want to mash or blend the baked meatballs and then add enough sauce to make it into the consistency of applesauce.

Chicken Meatballs in Orange Sweet and Sour Sauce

What to Use

Meatballs:
- Chicken (1 pound, ground lean)
- Egg (1 large, lightly beaten)
- Reduced-sodium soy sauce (2 tablespoons)
- Japanese Panko crumbs (.25 cup)
- Garlic (4 cloves, minced)
- Ginger (1 tablespoon, grated)
- Red onion (.25 cup, chopped)
- Cilantro (.5 cup, chopped, fresh)
- Sea salt (.25 teaspoon)
- Black pepper (.25 teaspoon)
- Dark sesame oil (1 tablespoon)

Orange Sauce:
- Orange juice (1 cup, fresh)
- Sugar-free ketchup (.25 cup)
- Agave nectar (.25 cup)
- Reduced-sodium soy sauce (.25 cup)
- Rice vinegar (2 tablespoons)
- Cornstarch (2 tablespoons)

What to Do

- Preheat oven to 450 degrees Fahrenheit. Line a jelly-roll pan with foil, and put it into the oven.
- Blend until finely chopped the garlic, ginger, red onion and cilantro. Put into a bowl.
- Add the beaten eggs, soy sauce, salt and pepper, Panko crumbs and the chicken to the chopped veggies in the bowl. Mix together with washed hands until well mixed. Chill for 30 minutes.
- Form into meatballs with a diameter of one inch.
- Heat up the oil in a large skillet to medium-high heat. Brown the meatballs in the skillet on both sides.
- Take the pre-heated jelly-roll pan out of the oven. Place the browned meatballs in the pan in one layer and return the pan to the oven. Bake for 20 minutes (at the same 450 degrees F).
- Meanwhile, mix together the sauce ingredients and heat the sauce on the stove over medium-high heat until it boils. Reduce the heat and let the sauce simmer uncovered for 2-3 minutes or until thickened.
- When you are off of your diet, you could just roll each meatball in the sauce after the meat balls are baked through and eat them that way. But while you are in the second stage of your post-surgery diet, you'll want to mash or blend the baked meatballs and then add enough sauce to make it into the consistency of applesauce.

Cheesy Turkey Meatballs in Marinara Sauce

What to Use
- Turkey (1.5 pounds, ground, fat-free)
- Italian-seasoned turkey sausage (.5 pound, casings removed)
- Italian-style bread crumbs (.25 cup)
- Low-fat milk (2 tablespoons)
- Egg (1, slightly beaten)
- Sea salt (.5 teaspoon)
- Black pepper (.5 teaspoon, freshly ground)
- Mozzarella cheese (8 ounces, cut into 17 small pieces)
- Marinara pasta sauce (one 26-ounce jar)

What to Do
- Preheat oven to 350 degrees Fahrenheit. Line a baking sheet with some parchment paper.
- In a bowl, mix the turkey, turkey sausage, bread crumbs, beaten egg, milk, salt and pepper with your (washed) hands.
- Shape the meat mixture into about 17 meatballs that are about golf ball size.
- Place the meatballs on the baking sheet. Press a deep hole in the middle of each one with your knuckle or finger. Place a small piece of cheese in each hole and close up the holes by pinching the meat together.
- Bake at 350 degree Fahrenheit for between 15 and 20 minutes or until done.
- Meanwhile, heat up the pasta sauce on the stove until bubbly hot.
- When you are off of your diet, you could just roll each meatball in the sauce after the meat balls are baked through and eat them that way. But while you are in the second stage of your post-surgery diet, you'll want to mash or blend the baked meatballs and then add enough sauce to make it into the consistency of applesauce.

Greek Quinoa Beef Meatballs

What to Use
- Ground beef (1 pound, extra-lean)
- Italian turkey sausage (.5 pound, casings removed)
- Red bell pepper (.5 of a pepper, seeds and membranes removed, sliced)
- Carrot (.5 cup, shredded)
- Garlic (2 cloves)
- Parsley leaves (2 tablespoons, fresh)
- Oregano leaves (2 tablespoons, fresh)
- Quinoa (1 cup cooked, from .5 cup dry)
- Feta cheese crumbles (one 5-ounce container)
- Sea salt (.5 teaspoon)
- Black pepper (.25 teaspoon, freshly grounded)
- Feta Dill Greek Yogurt Salad Dressing (6 ounces, OPA by Litehouse TM)

What to Do

- Preheat oven to 350 degrees Fahrenheit. Line baking sheet with parchment paper. Set aside.
- Cook the quinoa.
- Blend the red bell pepper, garlic, carrot, oregano and parsley to the fineness you need.
- In a bowl, combine the cooked quinoa with the blended veggies. Add the turkey sausage, ground beef, cheese, salt and pepper. Mix together good.
- Use a melon baller or your hands to make 32 meatballs, and place meatballs on the baking sheet.
- Bake at 350 degrees F for between 15 and 18 minutes or until cooked through.
- When you are off of your diet, you could just roll each meatball in the yogurt salad dressing (perhaps mixed with chopped cucumbers) and wrap in butter lettuce leaves after the meat balls are baked through and eat them that way. But while you are in the second stage of your post-surgery diet, you'll want to mash or blend the baked meatballs and then add enough sauce to make it into the consistency of applesauce.

Slow Cooker Pulled Pork in BBQ Sauce

What to Use

Meatballs:
- Boneless pork roast (one 2 to 3 pound roast)
- Onion (1 medium, thinly sliced)
- Garlic (3 medium cloves, thinly sliced)
- Chicken broth (1 cup)
- Sugar-free brown sugar (1 tablespoon)
- Chili powder (1 tablespoon)
- Sea salt (2 teaspoons)
- Cumin (.5 teaspoon, ground)
- Cinnamon (.5 teaspoon, ground)

BBQ Sauce:
- Liquid smoke (1 tablespoon)
- Sugar-free brown sugar (2 tablespoons)
- Worcestershire sauce (2 tablespoons)
- Reduced-sodium soy sauce (.25 cup)
- Beef broth (1 cup)
- Sugar-free ketchup (2 cups)

What to Do

- Put the onions and the garlic into your slow cooker in one even layer. Pour the broth over them.
- In a bowl, mix together sugar, cinnamon, cumin, salt, and chili powder.
- Use paper towels to pat the pork dry.
- Rub the pork all over with the spice mixture. Put the coated pork on top of the onions and garlic in the slow cooker. Cover.
- Cook on low for 8-10 hours or cook on high for 4-6 hours.
- While you are in stage two of your post-gastric sleeve operation diet, you'll need to let the cooked meat, onions and garlic cool a little and then blend it all in your blender. Put into a storage container. Take out the amount you need, add enough sauce to make it the consistency of applesauce, and heat it up whenever you want to eat some of it.
- To make the sauce, put all ingredients for the BBQ sauce in a large skillet and heat over medium heat.

Chapter 7:
Follow the Rules and Watch for Medical Complications

Continual weight loss, including fat

You likely had your surgery because you need to lose weight. If that is the case, the fat remains for now because only part of your stomach was removed, not any fat.

The good news is that research studies show that people who have this kind of surgery lose more than half of their excess weight! The successful people are the ones who follow the recommended dietary plan and keep their follow-up medical appointments.

Here are two rules to keep in mind:

Don't overeat - Even though your stomach is now smaller, it is possible to stretch it out by overeating. If you allow that to happen, your surgery will have been in vain and you will not lose weight.

Stay away from the sweets – This has been mentioned several times now, but it is important to stay away from sugar if you want to lose the weight. Sugar is addicting, too. You will need to cut out high-calorie liquids, such as fruit juice or sodas unless consumed only occasionally, so that you will lose the weight.

Weight loss will be achieved through the combination of eating less food than you did before your surgery (but now you will feel full sooner) and eating only nutritious quality food from here on out.

Prevention and/or awareness of possible EARLY medical problems

There are several complications that you need to watch out for. The early complications occur during your operation or within the following 30 days. The late complications occur after you are 30 days out from surgery.

While there are several possible problems that can be caused or aggravated by having the gastric sleeve surgery, you can prevent the onset of nutritional deficiency through juicing and consuming particular powerful plants using the recipes that are contained in this book.

Bleeding – Bleeding from the staple line itself should stop within a short period of time, but an injured spleen should have been removed at the time of the surgery to control bleeding going forward. Also, bleeding could come from blood vessels that surround the stomach, which cannot be allowed to continue. If you bleed out too much, you will need a blood transfusion.

Staple Leak - If a leak forms in the stomach that allows food and drink to get into the abdominal cavity, an infection that is called peritonitis can form. If peritonitis forms, it will need immediate medical attention because it can quickly become life-threatening.

Symptoms of peritonitis are rapid breathing, chills and fever, a rapid pulse, nausea and vomiting, swelling of the abdomen, and/or severe pain in the abdomen that sometimes reaches the shoulders and gets worse when you move, press on it or cough. Fortunately, only about 1% of gastric sleeve patients get it.

One thing you can do to prevent leakage of food into the abdomen is to prevent the stitches from tearing. To keep them from tearing, you need to take care that you do not do any heavy lifting and that you do not get constipated.

Avoid *lifting heavy things or doing strenuous exercise* if you had open surgery until your stomach heals. If you allow yourself to get *constipation*, it may cause you to strain yourself on the toilet, tearing your stitches up in your stomach. Keep your stools soft with the recommended soft foods, liquified food, and plenty of water.

The healing process will likely take four to six weeks. If your surgery was done by laparoscopic procedure, it will take less time than that to heal.

Deep Vein Thrombosis - A pulmonary embolism, which is a blood clot in one of your lungs, can form. An artery in the lung gets blocked by a blood clot (thrombosis) that was in a leg vein and broke loose and traveled to the lung area. Odd as this may sound, this is a risk of having gastric sleeve surgery.

This only affects between .5 and 2% of gastric sleeve patients. Taking blood thinners prior to surgery and afterwards from three months to a year (or even indefinitely) is advisable if you know that you have a deep vein thrombosis that could dislodge during or after your gastric surgery.

Wound infection – Infection at the site of the incision could form, especially if the procedure was performed openly. Treat these with local wound care and a change of dressings. Antibiotics are sometimes required to knock it out.

Death – Only one person in 400 people dies from complications that arise from having this surgery, but it is good to take all precautions.

Prevention and/or awareness of possible LATE medical problems

Difficulty swallowing and persistent reflux – These happen if the sleeve is too narrow, making it hard for the food to get into the stomach and on through it and also aggravating an existing reflux condition. The sleeve needs to be dilated if you find yourself in one of these situations. Meanwhile, consume only food that you can swallow and process.

Nutrition deficiency, leading to osteoporosis and anemia - Your doctor or his dietitian likely gave you some suggestions for things to eat that would provide you with protein, vitamins and minerals. Since your stomach is much smaller now, you need to make sure that you only put quality food in it from now on.

Our food supply is stripped of many of the nutrients that it used to have in days gone by, so eating less food, even if it is the most nutritious food that is commonly available, will put you in danger of becoming malnourished.

Therefore, you will need to take supplements from now on in addition to proper eating so as to make sure that you get all of the nutrition that your body will need. The dangers of not getting sufficient nutrients include osteoporosis and anemia.

Gallstones - Gallstones develop in some people who have the surgery that you just underwent because of rapid weight loss. These stones form in the bile ducts (the tubes that carry your bile to your small intestine) or in the gallbladder.

They would only cause you problems and pain if they block the opening to your gallbladder. If you have one attack, you will have more if you don't get surgery for it.

Hernia – If your surgery is open, your chances of getting hernias at the sites of incision are much higher than if it was performed laparoscopically. Obesity and diabetes also increase your chances of getting a hernia.

Regaining weight – You need to commit to your new lifestyle proper diet and exercise if you are to successfully keep the weight off. Statistics show that patients regain between 5 and 10% of the weight they lost initially. The sleeves dilate, so it is possible to stretch your sleeve, accommodating more food and failing to permanently lose the weight.

Conclusion

Thank you again for downloading this book!

I hope this book was able to help you to plan for your liquid and soft food post-operation meals.

The next steps are to make out your grocery shopping list, try a few of the recipes out, and then make some of them ahead of time (the ones that would taste good thawed) and freeze them.

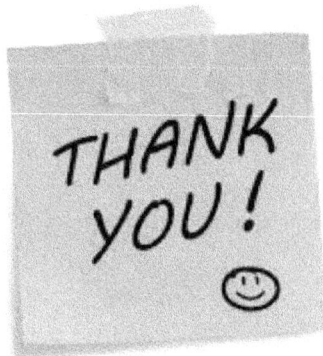

Gastric Sleeve Diet

Step By Step Guide For Planning What to Do and Eat Before and After Your Surgery

© Copyright 2017 by John Carter - All rights reserved.

This document is geared towards providing exact and reliable information in regards to the topic and issue covered. The publication is sold on the idea that the publisher is not required to render the accounting, officially permitted, or otherwise, qualified services. If advice is necessary, legal or professional, a practiced individual in the profession should be ordered.

- From a Declaration of Principles which was accepted and approved equally by a Committee of the American Bar Association and a Committee of Publishers and Associations.

In no way is it legal to reproduce, duplicate, or transmit any part of this document by either electronic means or in printed format. Recording of this publication is strictly prohibited and any storage of this document is not allowed unless with written permission from the publisher. All rights reserved.

The information provided herein is stated to be truthful and consistent, in that any liability, in terms of inattention or otherwise, by any usage or abuse of any policies, processes, or directions contained within is the solitary and utter responsibility of the recipient reader. Under no circumstances will any legal responsibility or blame be held against the publisher for any reparation, damages, or monetary loss due to the information herein, either directly or indirectly.

Respective authors own all copyrights not held by the publisher.

The information herein is offered for informational purposes solely and is universal as so. The presentation of the information is without a contract or any type of guarantee assurance.

The trademarks that are used are without any consent, and the publication of the trademark is without permission or backing by the trademark owner. All trademarks and brands within this book are for clarifying purposes only and are the owned by the owners themselves, not affiliated with this document.

Bonus:

FREE Report Reveals The Secrets To Lose Weight

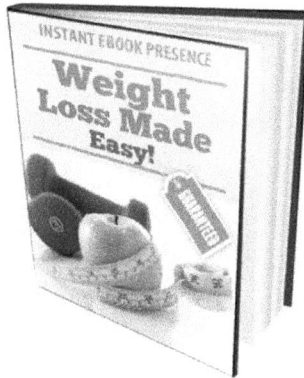

Weight loss doesn't happen from dieting only. Diets are short term solutions to shed extra weight. Diets do not work in the long term because people hate being on a diet (it's ok, you can admit that here). The only long term solution for permanent weight loss is to create new eating habits. This doesn't mean that chocolate will never pass your lips again, but it does mean looking after yourself and watching what you eat...

You can lose weight when you have the right reasons and motivation, and a part of this guide is to help you to find the motivation you need to change your weight...

Go to Get This Guid For FREE

http://www.sportsforsoul.com/weight-loss-2/

Table Of Contents:

Introduction

I want to thank you and congratulate you for downloading the book, *"Gastric Sleeve Diet Guide: Planning What to Do and Eat Before and After Your Surgery"*. This book gives an overall, but detailed, view of the various aspects regarding the patient's experience with gastric sleeve surgery.

Gastric sleeve surgery is compared to gastric bypass surgery so that the reader can be confident that the gastric sleeve procedure is the right choice for them. Various risks associated with each procedure, though not likely, are discussed.

Proven steps and strategies on various things the gastric sleeve patient needs to do and eat before their surgery are discussed. Emphasis is made on how to find the correct surgeon for you. Many common questions that gastric sleeve patients have are answered in this book, including the subjects of stomach stretching and pain.

Common diets for the two-week period before the surgery and for the various time periods following the surgery are given, as well as the reasons the patient needs to stay on the surgeon's prescribed diet. Recipes are not included in this book.

Every effort was made to give the reader the information that he needs to plan a course to safely reach his or her weight loss goal through the use of the gastric sleeve procedure.

Thanks again for downloading this book. I hope you enjoy it!

Chapter 1: Be Sure About Your Procedure Choice

What Gastric Sleeve Surgery is

The other name for this procedure is *sleeve gastrectomy*. It is a *restrictive operation* that makes your stomach smaller so that you will feel fuller quicker and eat less food. This procedure involves the removal of more than half of your stomach. After your surgery, only a vertical tube that is about the size of a banana is left.

This surgery should be considered as a tool for weight loss rather than a quick fix because the patient will need to eat a healthy diet and exercise following the surgery. It is <u>not</u> cosmetic surgery where fat is removed. Only part of the stomach is removed.

History

United Healthcare (insurance) added sleeve gastrectomy to their list of surgeries that they cover for weight loss on January 1, 2010. Almost all other major health insurance companies began to cover this procedure during the next two years.

It is extremely difficult to get health insurance companies to approve new procedures, but gastric sleeve surgery was approved because there was evidence that the procedure brought about significant weight loss and the complication rates were low.

Additionally, surgeons were already doing the procedure on patients who were covered by insurance. This was an accomplishment because surgery on obese people is riskier than surgery on people of normal size.

The gastric sleeve procedure initially was the first of two surgeries that were normally done. Insurance companies paid for the first surgery and then paid for the second one a year or so later after weight was lost. However, it was discovered that the sleeve procedure was successful in getting people's weight off without the second surgery being done.

Sleeve patients lost as much weight as the gastric bypass patients did over time. The gastric sleeve procedure proved to be quicker, less complicated, and safer than the gastric bypass procedure, and the surgeons quickly started to prefer performing the sleeve operations.

Patients liked the results too because they just didn't experience hunger anymore. In fact, some of them had to remind themselves to eat.

Reasons for Gastric Sleeve Surgery

This surgery is done to help people to lose weight and to keep the extra weight off. This procedure is done when the patient is severely overweight and has been unable to lose weight through diet, exercise or medicine and where emotional eating was not the cause for the weight gain.

Even though the smaller stomach can eventually be stretched out to accommodate more food, this surgery encourages the patient to eat less food so that obesity won't remain a problem.

Candidates for this procedure have a body mass index that is 40 - 60 (or even higher) and/or they have a weight-related life-threatening or disabling problem and a body mass index of at least 35.

Studies show that obese people who undergo this surgery are less likely to die from cancer, diabetes and heart problems than obese people who never lose the weight.

The gastric sleeve procedure is less risky than a gastric bypass is because the small intestine is not divided and reconnected like it is in a bypass procedure. Major complications that require re-operation occur in less than 5% of gastric sleeve patients.

Even though the gastric sleeve surgery is now often the only gastric procedure that is performed on the patient, it is still sometimes done as part of a larger approach where this surgery is followed up with an intestinal rerouting procedure. The weight loss that occurs as a result of the first surgery often makes the second one unnecessary.

Sometimes a surgeon who goes into surgery planning to perform a gastric bypass procedure changes his mind during the operation in favor of performing a gastric sleeve procedure because of an enlarged liver or an extensive amount of scar tissue in the intestines that make a gastric bypass impossible.

Other reasons people get the gastric sleeve surgery include body severe comorbidities, Crohn's disease, advanced age, a need to surveil the stomach or to continue taking specific medications, or any combination of the above that increases risk for the patient if the bypass procedure were done.

To Get the Sleeve or a Bypass...That is the Question

Be sure that it is the gastric sleeve procedure that you want and not the gastric bypass procedure.

Even though it is the riskiest type of bariatric surgery, the gastric bypass procedure still accounts for about 80% of the bariatric procedures that are done in the United States. Laparoscopic adjustable gastric band and the gastric sleeve procedure make up the other 20%, perhaps because the sleeve is a relatively new procedure and not all surgeons know how to perform it.

If the sleeve procedure is done laparoscopically rather than by open surgery, it is sometimes referred to as a laparoscopic sleeve gastrectomy. The laparoscopic sleeve gastrectomy is a fairly new procedure, but it is growing in popularity.

Gastric bypass surgery - In the gastric bypass procedure, the intestines are bypassed. The shortened intestines give your body less time to absorb the calories. The stomach is also made smaller.

The power of this method is therefore twofold because the patient loses weight from a restricted size of their stomach (they eat less food) and from malabsorption of calories.

Additionally, eating junk food or eating too much food for the small capacity will make the person who has had this procedure very sick. You can read information about "dumping" below in the gastric bypass benefits section. Dumping undigested food into the small intestine makes the patient sick.

Gastric bypass surgery is recommended for people who have a body mass index that is over 45. The gastric bypass procedure makes the body lose 60 – 80% of the extra weight in just a year's time in and forces a change in eating habits.

Gastric sleeve surgery - Conversely, gastric sleeve patients only lose between 50 and 70 percent of it over twice the length of time - two years. However, patients who undergo this surgery do tend to catch up with the weight loss of the bypass procedure within three years and they appear better toned when they get there than bypass patients do because of losing the weight more gradually.

This surgery involves the removal of 70% of the stomach in the area where the hunger hormone is produced. Therefore, much of the weight-loss power of the gastric sleeve option is in the fact that the patient doesn't get very hungry.

Even though this surgery has been used as the first of two procedures that are done to obtain considerable weight loss, many surgeons find that many super-obese gastric sleeve patients lose a sufficient amount of weight following the gastric sleeve surgery to make the planned second surgery (to reroute the intestines) unnecessary.

Both the gastric bypass procedure and the gastric sleeve procedure can be done either laparoscopically or by open surgery, but laparoscopically is becoming ever more popular.

Laparoscopic Method – In this method, several small incisions are made in the abdomen, so it is much less invasive than the open method is. The surgery on the stomach is done using a camera to guide the surgeon and small instruments to perform the operation with. This method is becoming more and more popular.

Open Method – In open surgery, the surgeon makes a large incision, laying the patient open to be worked on in traditional fashion.

Both the gastric bypass and the gastric sleeve surgeries are permanent, so you need to be very sure about which procedure you want because you cannot reverse what is done in these two surgeries.

Factors to Consider – The decision to have a gastric sleeve surgery or a gastric bypass surgery depends on:

The <u>gastric sleeve benefits</u> over those of bypass

- Less complicated - The gastric sleeve procedure is less complicated than the bypass procedure is, so it is also less risky because the small intestine is not cut and then reconnected in this procedure as it is in the bypass procedure.

- Shorter operation time - The operation time for the gastric sleeve is shorter than the time it takes to do a bypass, which makes the sleeve a little safer.

- Works through hunger reduction - The gastric sleeve works through reducing hunger in the patient since 70% of the stomach area that produces the hunger hormone ghrelin is removed. Some patients have to remind themselves to eat for a half of a year after their surgery. The bypass procedure also reduces hunger a bit, but not as much as the sleeve procedure does.

- Slower rate of weight loss – It takes the body about 18 months to lose a massive amount of weight following a gastric sleeve procedure, which is slower than the loss that follows a bypass but faster than the lap band.

- Better appearance in the end - The slower pace of weight loss produces less saggy skin and fewer stretch marks than you would get with the super-fast weight loss that comes from the bypass procedure.

- Fewer vitamins required to be purchased for the remainder of life - You will need to buy fewer vitamins after this procedure than you will following the bypass surgery.

- Lower mortality rate - The mortality rate is lower from this procedure than it is from the bypass procedure, although it is below 1% for both procedures.

- Far less dumping episodes - The sleeve doesn't produce the dumping syndrome nearly as much as the bypass procedure does, so you won't get terribly sick should you eat something that is off of your diet. Sugar has time to digest. You may consider dumping to be a benefit of the bypass, however, since it prevents you from eating junk food for the rest of your life!

- No adjustments needed - Compared to the lap band, no adjustments are needed.

The gastric bypass benefits over those of the sleeve

- Long-established, well-known procedure - The bypass procedure has been around longer than the sleeve method and is considered "the gold standard." Laparoscopic surgeons have a lot of experience in the gastric bypass procedure.

- Few calories absorbed - Since much of the intestines are

bypassed and the used part is short, you don't consume as many calories as you do if the full length of the intestines is used.

- Lowers GERD risk - The gastric bypass lowers your risk of acid reflux (GERD), so your surgeon will likely recommend you opt for the bypass if you have a history of acid reflux.

- Big weight loss immediately - Gastric bypass patients lose between 60 and 80 percent of their excess body weight during the first year following their surgery. This massive weight loss happens because of the unpleasant experience of the *dumping syndrome* that occurs whenever the patient eats or drinks sugary or fatty (junk) food and drink.

  The dumping syndrome is a condition where undigested sweet or fatty foods pass through the stomach and into the small intestine rapidly, causing nausea, vomiting, diarrhea, cramping, dizziness and fatigue.

Some people view this dumping aspect of the bypass procedure to be a   positive thing rather than a negative thing because it forces them to eat better.

Dumping usually happens just 15 to 30 minutes after eating junk food. Late dumping happens after three hours and just makes people sweat and feel weak and dizzy. Some people experience both types of dumping.

Why we are not discussing lap band

Many surgeons who have a good amount of experience in lap band, sleeve gastrectomy and in gastric bypass surgeries have found that many of the people who get the lap band don't end up losing weight because the lap band patients often don't dedicate themselves to changing their diet and to exercising. *While patients who have the other procedures done must also change their lifestyle, the failure rate is much higher in lap band patients.*

Surgeons want their patients to succeed for both the patients' sake and for their own reputation. Patients who lose a lot of weight will likely refer other people to the surgeon. Surgeons cannot always determine which people will follow a new diet and exercise regimen and which ones will not.

Additionally, the lap band is a hassle for both the patient and the surgeon after a lap band is put into the patient's body because the patient must go back to the surgeon several times per year for the rest of the patient's life to get the band fill levels checked. With a sleeve or a bypass operation, no foreign object has been inserted, and the patient is done with the surgeon after a few check-ups.

How long the surgery would be for gastric sleeve versus gastric bypass

It is always risky to be under anesthesia. It is even higher for obese people to be under anesthesia. High cholesterol and high blood pressure increase the risks even more. While procedural time is a minor factor in making your decision, but it should still be considered when the risk is highest.

The average surgery time for a *gastric sleeve* operation is only 1 hour and 40 minutes, but the average surgery time for a *gastric bypass* operation is 2 hours and almost 45 minutes.

How fast I will lose weight after gastric sleeve versus gastric bypass

As previously stated, weight loss from *gastric bypass* is greater from the start in comparison to *gastric sleeve* surgery, however, weight loss after the gastric sleeve begins to catch up within three years after the surgery. The slower weight loss time following the gastric sleeve surgery also produces less saggy skin and fewer stretch marks. Still, some people prefer to get skinny quickly.

Body mass index affects the speed of weight loss too because the higher the patient's initial body mass index, the more weight they lose, no matter which method is used.

Chapter 2: Compare Sleeve Complications to Bypass Complications

There are several more complications associated with the gastric bypass procedure than with the gastric sleeve procedure. You should take a look at what the complications are with each option, especially if you are still not sure which procedure to have.

Sleeve	Bypass	
Gastroesophageal Reflux Disease (GERD)	X	
Staple line failure (then infection, abscess...)	X	
Stricture (chronic)	X	
Stricture (acute)	X	X
Nutritional deficiencies	X	X
Gallstones	X	X
Venous thromboembolism	X	X
Death	X	X
Nausea		X
Dehydration		X
Indigestion		X
Reactive hypoglycemia		X
Incisional hernia		X

Wound infection	X
Marginal ulcers	X
Stomal stenosis (Stricture)	X
Anastomotic leaks	X
Hemorrhage	X

Gastroesophageal Reflux Disease (GERD)

With risk as high as 47%, GERD is a very common complication that *gastric sleeve* patients experience. It starts off with occasional episodes of gastroesophageal reflux and heartburn. As time goes on, the esophagus structure changes and the patient gets inflammation of the esophagus for which the patient takes proton pump inhibitors.

Staple Line Failure

This complication is one that surgeons try to prevent. Special attention is given to putting staples into the stomach where the stomach is reattached to itself.

In a staple line failure, food and drink get through this area, getting into the abdominal cavity. When food and drink get into the abdominal cavity, an infection called peritonitis sets in, which can become life-threatening.

Symptoms include a rapid heart rate, chills, fever, nausea, vomiting, swelling of the abdomen, rapid breathing, and/or severe pain.

If it happens within a week following the gastric sleeve surgery, a laparoscopy may be attempted to locate and repair the leaking area. If the leak happens after a week, the area is drained and washed out, etc. The risk of line failure is 2.4%.

Stricture (chronic)

Chronic stricture is a complication that is associated with *gastric sleeve* surgery, and it is the narrowing of the stomach outlet area at the place where it is attached surgically to the small bowel. With this condition, the patient has trouble eating solid food, has increased saliva and/or mucus, and also has reflux symptoms.

Stricture can happen after a month or two following your surgery. Sometimes it resolves itself in time. If it doesn't resolve itself, the treatment options depend on how long the narrow portion is. Endoscopic dilation is used when the narrowed portion is short. If the narrowed portion is long, repeated endoscopic dilation may be performed so as to fix the problem. If repeated dilation fails, the patient may then get the gastric bypass done.

Stricture (acute)

This condition more commonly follows *gastric bypass* surgery, but it sometimes happens to *gastric sleeve* patients.

Acute stricture is an acute narrowing of the stomach outlet area at the place where it is attached surgically to the small bowel. With this condition, the opening is so narrow that the patient even has trouble getting liquids through. The patient also experiences increased saliva and/or mucus, and reflux symptoms.

This can happen after a month or two following your surgery. Treatment involves replacing food and liquids with IV fluids and endoscopic dilation. There is a 3.5% risk for getting either a chronic or acute stricture following (usually bypass) surgery.

Nutritional deficiencies

Malnutrition is possible in both *gastric sleeve* and *gastric bypass* patients, especially if the supplements are not taken. Deficiencies for which you will need to compensate for with supplements for the rest of your life following your gastric surgery include the following:

Iron – Iron is needed for red blood cell production, for liver parenchymal cells, and for the reticuloendothelial system. Iron deficiency anemia will occur if supplements are not taken, especially in women of reproductive age who are menstruating.

Calcium and *Vitamin D* – A reduction in calcium, vitamin D and exercise will eventually result in bone resorption and osteoporosis.

Vitamin B12 – Deficiency in B12 results in emotional changes (depression, psychosis, and depression), decreased thinking capabilities, poor muscle function, changes in reflexes, low red blood cells, decreased fertility, reduced heart function, inflammation of the tongue and decreased taste.

Folate – This B vitamin makes and repairs DNA and produces red blood cells. A deficiency of this vitamin results in anemia, which deprives your tissues of oxygen and then affects their function. Birth defects are sometimes caused by folate deficiency during pregnancy. Folate deficiency symptoms include growth problems, tongue swelling, mouth sores, gray hair and fatigue. Folate deficiency leads to anemia, which has the symptoms of irritability, shortness of breath, pale skin, lethargy, weakness and persistent fatigue. Fortified cereals, fruits and vegetables contain folate.

Vitamin A – Night blindness is caused by lack of vitamin A in the diet, as is a diminished ability to fight off infections and maternal mortality.

Vitamin E – Deficiency in vitamin E causes neurological and neuromuscular problems, anemia, retinopathy and impairment of the immune response.

Vitamin K – A lack of vitamin K can result in massive uncontrolled bleeding, bleeding at the surgical sites, stomach pains, cartilage calcification, and malformation of developing bone. This vitamin in used by the liver to create enzymes needed for coagulation of the blood.

Selenium – Insufficient selenium results in muscle wasting, muscle myopathy, arrhythmia, cardiomyopathy, reduced thyroid, and immunity function. Loss of hair and skin pigment can also occur, along with encephalopathy and white nail beds. Absorption of selenium is helped along with vitamins C and E.

Protein – Protein prevents hair loss, sickness, flaky dermatitis, and fluid retention in the ankles and feet. Protein keeps bones, skin, nails, and hair healthy. Malabsorption can also lead to kidney oxalate stones and lactic acidosis.

Most importantly for the gastric sleeve patient, protein aids in proper wound healing and promotes weight loss. Protein helps with weight loss several ways.

- It satisfies and therefore discourages a dieter from eating extra calories due to hunger. Protein helps a person to feel full, strong and energized because protein takes longer to digest than carbs and some other foods do.

- The presence of protein ensures that it is fat and not metabolism-boosting muscle the body uses for fuel. If a person does not get enough protein, the body breaks down muscles to get what it needs. A person needs at least 50 and 60 grams of protein daily to prevent the loss of body muscle mass.

- Additionally, protein food requires the body to burn more calories to process than other kinds of food do.

Because the stomach of a gastric sleeve patient is small, protein needs to be consumed first so that the patient doesn't become too full to eat or drink protein. Both plant and animal sources of protein are needed in the food that is eaten.

Smoothies and shakes made with protein powders and other proper ingredients are useful for delivering a lot of protein in a small amount of drink, which is especially helpful in the first few weeks following a gastric sleeve surgery. Some people also take liquid protein supplements.

Men need between 70 and 90 grams of protein and women need between 60 and 80 grams of protein daily. The risk of protein deficiency in the gastric sleeve patient is about 12%.

Gallstones

Gallstones affect both *gastric sleeve* and *gastric bypass* patients. The risk of getting this complication is as high as 23% in people who lose a large amount of weight, but they are only a problem if they block the opening to the gallbladder. Bile salts prevent them from forming in the bile ducts or in the gallbladder, but the surgery causes malabsorption or the bile salts. If you have an attack, you will need to have surgery for it because it won't go away on its own.

Venous Thromboembolism

This condition is much more common in *gastric bypass* patients than in *gastric sleeve* patients, but it does occur following either procedure. The risk for this problem, whether a deep vein thrombosis or a pulmonary embolism, is less than one percent in gastric sleeve patients.

Death

It is possible to die from complications that arise following *either* one of these two gastric procedures.

Nausea

Nausea commonly follows *gastric bypass* surgery, but not gastric sleeve surgery. This condition is helped by following the diet that the patient's doctor or nutritionist recommends following the operation. A large amount of IV fluid will also help to alleviate nausea. The risk for this complication is 70% for the bypass patient.

Dehydration

Depletion of fluids is common in *gastric bypass* patients, but not in gastric sleeve patients. The risk is as high as 65% for bypass patients. Dehydration is resolved by drinking two liters of fluids per day. Vomiting and further dehydration occur if the bypass patient does not drink enough water. An IV line may be necessary if the dehydration gets bad enough.

Indigestion

Indigestion is a complication of *gastric bypass* surgery (but not gastric sleeve surgery), affecting 60% of patients. It can be defined as digestion difficulty that is accompanied by discomfort or burning in the upper abdomen.

It is helped by the avoidance of greasy food or possibly drinking only liquids for a while. H2 blockers and antacids are used if dietary changes don't solve the problem.

Reactive Hypoglycemia

Reactive hypoglycemia sometimes follows *gastric bypass* surgery, but not gastric sleeve surgery, and it happens between

45 and 60 minutes after a patient who has a low blood sugar eats a high-carbohydrate meal. It also often occurs because of the excessive "dumping" of undigested food into the small intestines that happens in bypass patients.

The person gets lightheaded, sweaty and their heart rate increases because of the imbalance between insulin and blood sugar in the bloodstream. Insulin that remains after blood sugar is used causes low blood sugar.

To resolve the situation, the patient needs to drink two ounces of skim milk or a few ounces of diluted juice. This condition can be prevented by eating proteins first and avoiding the consumption of sugar. Additionally, medications are sometimes prescribed to manage the condition. Part of the pancreas is removed in extreme situations so as to manage this condition. The risk for reactive hypoglycemia is only 1%.

Incisional Hernia

An Incisional hernia sometimes follows *gastric bypass* surgery, but not usually gastric sleeve surgery. An incisional hernia is an opening that forms when an internal body part or organ comes out through a surgical incision because of the incision not healing correctly. This is a dangerous condition because the intestine becomes obstructed.

This kind of hernia occurs in 20% of patients who have an open surgical procedure and in only 0.2% of patients who have laparoscopic procedures, and they show up several months after the procedure.

Wound Infection

Wound infection sometimes follows *gastric bypass* surgery, but not gastric sleeve surgery. Bacteria are released from the bowel while the stomach is being operated on, infecting the incisions. Sometimes the inside of the abdomen is what get infected. Additionally, kidney and bladder infections can occur.

Physical activity, respiratory therapy, and, of course, antibiotics after surgery can lower the risk of infection. The risk level of wound infection is 12%, with the vast majority occurring in patients who underwent open surgery instead of laparoscopic surgery.

Marginal Ulcers

Marginal ulcers sometimes follow *gastric bypass* surgery, but not gastric sleeve surgery. A new stomach pouch is created when a person undergoes gastric bypass surgery and this kind of ulcer most commonly forms in the new pouch. A burning pain in the stomach is common to ulcer sufferers.

Proper dietary habits and the avoidance of smoking and NSAIDs help the bypass patient to avoid getting marginal ulcers. Endoscopy can be performed to confirm their presence, but their treatment is usually just antacids. The risk factor for getting this is 12%.

Stomal Stenosis (Stricture)

Stomal stenosis sometimes follows *gastric bypass* surgery, but not usually following gastric sleeve surgery, although it can. It results from the buildup of scar tissue. This condition involves inflammation or blockage of the opening to or from the stomach, which prevents food from entering the stomach or intestines. It can be chronic or acute.

Symptoms include food intolerance, nausea, vomiting, and dysphagia. It is treated by fasting and hydration by IV. A second plan is an endoscopic dilation. The risk for this is 8%.

Anastomotic Leaks

Anastomotic leaks sometimes follow *gastric bypass* surgery, but not gastric sleeve surgery. This leak happens during surgery and is when digestive contents get into the abdomen when a connection is being made. It can be fixed if found quickly enough but can become infected if it is not found. A dye is used to see if the connection is secure. The risk factor is 5%.

Hemorrhage (bleeding)

Hemorrhages sometimes follow *gastric bypass* surgery, but not gastric sleeve surgery. Bleeding that sometimes follows bypass surgery include vomiting blood (hematemesis) or blood in the stools (melena stools). The risk for one of these is 3.2%.

Chapter 3: Ten Crucial Steps to Take Before Your Gastric Sleeve Surgery

Okay, now that you are sure about your decision to get the sleeve gastrectomy, there are some things that you need to think about and to do before you go in for your surgery. Here are some steps that you need to take.

Step One: Find out whether or not you qualify for a gastric sleeve surgery.

If you want to have weight loss surgery in the United States, there are some particular requirements that the National Institute of Health (NIH) says that you need to meet. You need to 1) be over 18 years old, and 2) have a body mass index of 40 or more or have a body mass index of 35 and one or more comorbid conditions.

The body mass index is a measurement of height over weight. Comorbid conditions are diseases that result from being overweight or are strongly related to being overweight. These conditions include, but are not limited to, soft tissue infections, venous stasis disease, type 2 diabetes, high cholesterol, high blood pressure, sleep apnea and arthritis.

Step Two: Find out whether or not your insurance will cover weight loss surgery.

Although you must be morbidly obese, being morbidly obese does not mean your insurance will cover the surgery. That is a separate thing you need to pursue. The insurance companies require what the NHI requires and often more.

The aforementioned conditions are usually covered by insurance. Sometimes an insurance company will also cover acid reflux disease, psychosocial stress resulting from obesity, stroke or risk of stroke, depression, gallbladder disease, fatty liver syndrome and/or congestive heart failure.

Visit ObesityCoverage.com to use their insurance checker tool.

Step Three: Find two potential surgeons.

To find a couple of potential surgeons, you will have to research, get onto some online forums, and possibly ask around.

Step Four: Attend a seminar.

Once you have a couple of candidates for a good surgeon, you need to learn some things from them. Surgeons usually have a way that you can register on their website to attend an in-person seminar. Sometimes an online seminar is available too.

Step Five: Set up a consultation with one or more of the surgeons you selected.

After you learn general things from the seminar's information, you'll likely have some questions for the surgeon that you select to perform your operation. Set up and attend a consultation with the surgeon. Have those questions ready to ask him. See the Frequently Asked Questions information for what questions you might want to ask.

Step Six: Obtain a Letter of Medical Necessity from your primary care physician.

Get your regular doctor to write for you a Letter of Medical Necessity to clear you for surgery.

Step Seven: Obtain insurance pre-approval for you to have the operation.

The surgeon's office will turn in your paperwork for you, but you need to call them from time to time to keep on top of where things stand.

Step Eight: Get the psychiatric tests and lab work done and obtain a medically supervised diet.

The surgeon will refer you to local providers who will administer the various tests.

Step Nine: Choose a surgery date. Make plans to be off of work for a while.

After you are approved for the surgery, choose a surgery date. Make plans to be off of work for at least two weeks. You won't want to lift heavy things, so judge the situation for yourself and allow yourself adequate time to heal properly.

Step Ten: Keep yourself focused, motivated and engaged in the process.

Get yourself involved in your own weight loss project, doing whatever that means for you. For example, you could study the experiences of other people and gather recipes for protein shakes, pureed food, and soft food that you think you might enjoy and try some of the recipes. Shop for food. Pre-make and freeze shakes (minus the ice) and other foods. You could get your helpers lined up, get ahead of the household laundry, cleaning, and other chores, including buying your vitamins and medicines, etc. Get excited and move things forward!

Chapter 4: Choosing the Right Surgeon for You

How do I choose a bariatric surgeon?

A local surgeon may be important to you because you will have to go see your surgeon several times before the surgery and several times after the surgery. Isolation often results in failed weight loss.

If the surgeon is not local, flying for the many visits you'll need to take is not a good option. Ask various surgeons how they accommodate out-of-town patients in things like recommendations for post-op visits, hotels, and whether or not you can check in without having to travel.

Research surgeons and their support staff through various methods. You can read about various surgeons online. You can read what others have to say in the various online support groups. You can ask acquaintances about surgeons they may have heard of or had experience with.

You want your surgeon to have credentials, so you will want him to:
- Be fellowship-trained as a bariatric surgeon
- Be board-certified in general surgery
- Participate in groups like the American Society of Metabolic and Bariatric Surgeons
- Participate in continuing education in bariatric surgery
- Have the support staff and adequate aftercare resources for you
- Have adequate experience performing gastric sleeve operations in the method you have chosen (laparoscopic or open)

You may want to meet some of his previous patients. You want to be able to trust the surgeon to meet your needs, listen to your concerns, answer your questions, give excellent care after the surgery, and offer various kinds of support

You may want to have your gastric sleeve surgery performed at a specialized hospital, one that is a Center of Excellence in bariatric surgery. Center of Excellence is a designation that says that the facility has:

- Has achieved excellence in their surgeries
- Has performed a specific minimum number of bariatric procedures during the prior year
- Staff that has taken extra training in weight loss surgery
- A bariatric coordinator who ensures that things run smoothly, often serving as the patient's main point of contact

You can find a Center of Excellence on the MBSAQIP (Metabolic and Bariatric Surgery Accreditation and Quality Improvement Program) website. Then you can choose from among the surgeons who practice there and make your surgeon selection that way. Don't rule out regular hospitals, however.

What do I ask the bariatric surgeon?

Once you have narrowed down a few surgeons and a hospital or two, you want a consultation with one or more surgeons, ask the questions listed below and any other questions you need answers to. Then select a surgeon.

> 1.) *Ask him about his surgery experience.* Ten years of experience is a respectable amount of experience with surgery and assures that he can handle any difficulties.

Even though having a lot of experience is desirable, the experience is not the same thing as skill. Some younger surgeons, even ones just coming out of a quality training program, can do a good job. They are likely in a two-year fellowship program where they specialize in a type of surgery.

Remember that the gastric sleeve procedure is one of the newer gastric procedures, so nobody has long-term experience with it. Fortunately, the gastric sleeve surgery is simpler and less risky than the bypass surgery procedure is and quickly gained the confidence of health insurance companies.

You also want to know specifically what his experience is with the particular method he plans to use on you, i.e. laparoscopic surgery vs. open surgery.

2.) *Ask the surgeon what resources he offers before and after the surgery.* Your weight loss success depends on more than just having had the operation. You will need to change how you eat and start to exercise too, so it would be useful to you if the surgeon has some resources available that would support you while you go on the weight loss journey. You need a good surgeon who also has a good bariatric coordinator and dietitian.

A dietician who listens to you and can work out a plan for you that is tailored to your situation would be a great resource. Some surgeons offer online support groups, weekly in-person support groups and/or Facebook support groups that discuss various subjects relating to life after bariatric surgery. Smartphone apps that keep you connected are also offered by some surgeons.

3.) *Ask the surgeon which procedures he performs.* Not all surgeons offer all procedures or know how to do all of them. Ask why they don't offer the one(s) they don't offer. If they push for one kind of surgery, they may have some sort of self-interest involved and you may benefit more from a different surgeon.

You likely have an enlarged liver. If it is too large, its size would prevent the sleeve procedure from being done laparoscopically because the doctor would not be able to push the liver far enough to the side to access your stomach. If the surgeon also knows how to do a sleeve gastrectomy using the open method or if he knows how to do the bypass surgery, there are more options available to get the job done while you are under anesthesia. You wouldn't want him to just sew you up having done nothing for lack of knowledge.

4.) *Ask the surgeon which procedure he recommends for you.* A good surgeon would know that one procedure is not the best fit for every person. A good surgeon will want to find out more about you before he answers the question. He'll need to know what you eat, how much you exercise, what your risk tolerances are, etc. If you do emotional eating or binge eating, he may suggest you get the bypass surgery instead of the sleeve procedure because the bypass procedure will force you to change your eating habits.

And actually, he would try to present you with the risks and the benefits associated with each procedure as they relate to you and let you decide.

Talk to your surgeon about your goals and about your fears. Be confident that you are making the right procedure choice and surgeon choice before you have a procedure done.

If he rushes through your consultation, your future experiences with him will likely also be rushed. You will see the surgeon several times before your surgery and a few times during the following year after your surgery, so you need to be able to benefit from your visits with him.

5.) *Ask the surgeon what his complication rates are.* These are complications that occur during or around the time of the operation. They do not include minor postoperative complications.

The national averages for complications during the various surgeries are 3.6% for gastric bypass, **2.2% for a gastric sleeve**, and just 0.9% for lap band procedures, so you want this surgeon's complication rate to be at or below the national average of 2.2% for gastric sleeve surgeries. Hopefully, he has enough surgeries under his belt (at least 100) so that it would be possible to get a truly representative percentage.

6.) *Ask the surgeon why you should select him to do the operation.* This will be an unusual question for a surgeon to receive, but if he can answer it with something about how he loves his job and will be supportive of you on your journey, you may be more comfortable with him than if he just brags about his skills.

Chapter 5: More Questions to Ask before Surgery

How much weight can I expect to lose?

You need to know how much weight you should expect to lose after the surgery. Do the calculations and you will know. You will lose somewhere around 60% of the extra weight over two years, with likely the majority of it coming off in the first year.

Long-term weight loss, however, is more dependent on what you eat, how much you exercise, etc. than on which one of the procedures you choose. It is possible to gain all of the weight back.

Will my stomach stretch after surgery?

It can stretch, but it depends on how much you normally feed it. For an occasional large meal, your stomach can stretch to accommodate it and then get back to its smaller size. However, if you continue to give it large meals (or meals too large for the size your stomach will be), then it can and will stretch and not get back to its smaller size. If you stretch it back out, you eat more food. When you eat more food, you gain weight.

People often become fat because their hunger and full signals are actually broken. It would be best to monitor how much food you eat. Even an occasional small sweet is better than an excessively large amount of quality food because you are not stretching your stomach.

Can I still drink alcohol after my gastric sleeve surgery?

Yes, you can have alcohol after your surgery, but it will make you drunker much faster than before you have your surgery because of having a smaller stomach that holds less food. It would be advisable to just give up alcohol.

While you can have wine or something after your surgery, you need to be very aware that one or two glasses of wine for you would have the same effect as six or seven glasses of wine would have on a person who has a normal-sized stomach. If you do that regularly, you become an alcoholic.

In fact, studies show that many people who have no history of alcohol abuse easily become alcoholics and get charged with DWIs from about two years after having a gastric sleeve surgery onward because they drink the same amount of alcohol they did before their surgery, not realizing the effect alcohol has on them after their stomach has become small.

Let your family know this if you drink at all so they can help you keep your alcohol consumption under control.

You also need to remember that alcohol is a carbohydrate as well as something that can make you drunk. As a carbohydrate, it has no nutritional benefit, and too much of it can cause you to gain weight. 'Too much" for a person with a small stomach is not very much.

Alcohol is also toxic to your body and will negatively affect your liver much faster than you would imagine it would. You will need to keep all of this information in mind if you must drink.

Besides sensitivities to alcohol, what other sensitivities might I expect as a result of having a smaller stomach?

You will be more sensitive to all carbohydrates and proteins consumed, as well as to the vitamins and minerals that you ingest.

In addition to food and drink, you will also be more sensitive to things that you smell. Chemicals and other odors may create responses that you did not have before you had your gastric surgery.

What can I expect in the way bowel movements after gastric sleeve surgery?

While you are on the liquid and pureed diets, the bowels won't have trouble, although pain medication can lead to some constipation. Follow the guidelines you will be given and you should be okay during those phases.

After you start to consume regular food, you can expect some changes in your bowel movements. Be prepared for more gas, occasional cramping, different smells than you are used to, and likely some constipation if you are not careful to include fiber and liquid in the diet.

After your gastric sleeve surgery, your metabolism will have slowed down due to consuming few calories. The combination of regular food, a slowed metabolism, and the effects of pain medication can create stools that are hard to pass. Of all times to not force things, after surgery is definitely not the time to force things.

Fluids and fiber in your diet should help to prevent a potential constipation problem. If you have ongoing problems with constipation, despite your efforts to avoid having a constipation problem, talk to your surgeon about it.

How much pain will I experience?

This question is hard to answer because of the different ways that people rate pain. Open surgery is quite painful and it also requires a longer hospital stay than does laparoscopic surgery.

The site of incision is where the pain comes from, which is the reason that laparoscopic surgery causes far less pain than open surgery does. If you follow the diet guidelines before surgery and get your liver smaller so that the surgeon can move it out of the way, your surgeon will be able to perform the much less painful laparoscopic procedure on you. Following those diet instructions helps both of you!

The upper left quadrant, which is under your rib cage, is the site where most of the pain comes from. The incision there is widened and stretched to get the part of the stomach that is being removed out. Muscle fibers tear in that area and bruising results. Even so, pain can be managed with pain medications for the first few days.

Surgery Day – You will wake up groggy and you won't have much pain at first because of the pain medication you were administered. You will feel general soreness wherever incisions were made. You may also be a little nauseated from the anesthesia at first.

Your surgeon may actually want you to get up and walk on this day to reduce the pain that the CO_2 caused during the surgery. It will be difficult to get out of the bed on this day because you will be sore. The rest of the day, you will be on your back with the bed slightly inclined upward.

Day One – You will notice the pain much more on this day because the anesthesia will have worn off. You will have pain medication, but you will be moving around a bit more on this day. They will have you use the IV pain medication less and use oral ones more. If you had your surgery laparoscopically, the pain will be bearable.

Your throat will still be sore, dry and swollen from the tube that was put down it while you were under anesthesia, but drinking a little water should help.

You will be rolled by wheelchair to Radiology for your swallow test. Your doctor will ask you about your pain level, remove your catheter, and make sure you are able to get up onto your feet. He'll also answer questions then. He will discharge you if you had your procedure done laparoscopically.

Day Two and Three – Your pain is still bearable if you had the laparoscopic procedure done. Days three through six will be your most painful days because you will be on your feet more often and turning your trunk to the side more than when you were in the hospital, but your doctor should have given you instructions for pain management for this period. Let your surgeon know if your pain is unbearable.

Week One – After a few days, life can be more normal, although pain can flare up any time you stand up from a seated position, twist your torso, or bend over for the next several weeks. All of that will go away in time, though.

Most people are still in too much pain to return to work during this week, though the pain is not severe. Getting into and out of a car and running errands will cause the most pain. Some people are too tired to return to work too.

Week Two to Month Three – You should not have much pain at all by the second month after surgery. You are likely off of pain medication. Contact your doctor if you are in nagging pain after two months.

Month Three to Six and Beyond – You should not notice pain hardly ever by this point. If you do, talk to the doctor. Gastric sleeve patients who have gone through the whole process and got the weight off say that the pain was worth it in the end.

What exactly is stomach stapling?

The stomach is literally stapled back together with a surgical staple gun when the surgeon performs either a gastric sleeve procedure or a gastric bypass.

The staples close in the shape of a "B" to both compress enough to not allow bleeding while also allowing the blood to flow through the holes of the B. Tissue can heal properly using this type of staple. Loading the wrong staple size for the thickness of tissue can cause leaks, however.

What happens to the staples?

The staples will stay in you forever because they are made of titanium. Even if they move from their original position, they won't cause problems. Additionally, they are not magnetic and will not set off any x-ray machines at airports or other places.

Am I ready to make changes?

You need to decide inside yourself that you like yourself and want to treat yourself good. Remember who you were before you got fat (if it hasn't been a lifetime thing). What made you, you? Remember how good you looked in normal sized clothes and how your appearance gave you some self-confidence and mobility to do more things.

Get a vision of the new you in your mind and focus on it frequently. Decide in your mind that from now on you will change your eating habits and also do more exercise. The surgery is just a tool to help you in your journey, but you only lose weight and keep it off through your own efforts to change your lifestyle.

What does gastric sleeve surgery cost?

There are costs associated with the surgery both before the surgery and after the surgery. Some of the after-surgery costs will remain for the rest of your life.

The nutritionist consultation price is negotiated before your visit. Consultations with a nutritionist range between $50.00 and $100.00 per visit, and you pay for them out of pocket.

Of course, you will buy the food, protein powders, clothing for various sizes, etc., before your surgery. If you don't have a blender, you'll likely need to buy one.

The price of gastric sleeve surgery itself is typically much less than the cost of a gastric bypass but slightly more than a gastric band surgery. Costs vary by state. Generally speaking, the procedure tends to be cheaper in the southern half of the United States than it is in the northern half. Fortunately, the costs have been coming down due to increased competition and demand for the surgery.

Costs for gastric sleeve surgery range *between $9,600 and $26,000 in the United States.* The cost for the procedure is most often quoted to be around $14,900, but *$16,800 is about the average price for it.*

These figures represent what it would cost you to pay for the procedure yourself. Insurance companies are charged more than this, however.

After your surgery, your follow-up visits with your surgeon are free. However, if you have complications, it will cost a lot of money to treat the complications.

Complications will be covered by insurance if the surgery was covered by insurance. They will be paid for by you if you paid for the surgery out of pocket. Wound site infections, which are caused by the surgeon, are usually paid for by the surgery center or hospital.

After your surgery, your new lifestyle will cost you some extra money in the following ways:

Quality food - Even though your stomach will be smaller, food will be more expensive because you will be eating better quality food.

Gym membership - You may get a gym membership.

Supplements – If you spend money on nothing else, you will need to spend money on supplements for the rest of your life so that you can function because you will be missing much of your stomach and will therefore not be able to absorb sufficient nutrients. Quality protein supplements alone can cost you more than $50.00 per month.

Clothing - You will have to keep buying new clothes as you keep losing weight if you don't have much of your old clothes or didn't buy some before your surgery. You may want to buy things at Goodwill or at yard sales until you reach your goal and plateau out.

Cosmetic surgery - You may have cosmetic surgery done to remove excess skin that may droop from your body. You can save up for that expense.

What do I need to do at home before my surgery?

Change your diet early – You need to start the protein liquid diet one or two weeks before you have your surgery. This is done to shrink your liver, and that will make the surgery safer for you.

Make out a different kind of grocery list – You need to have a lot of protein both before and after your surgery, so you will need to get familiar with some protein smoothie and shake recipes. They are made with protein powders which come in various flavors. You will need clear liquids before you can have the shakes and smoothies, so you'll need to also have broth, unsweetened juices, etc., on your shopping list and in your home.

Buy yourself some clothes (or dig out old ones) – Right after your surgery, you will want loose-fitting clothes and slippers. Then you will need to fit into various sizes of clothes as you lose weight while you also heal.

Stop smoking – Your surgeon will not perform the surgery if your body does not test as being smoke-free. That is because you will not recover as well as you would if you didn't have that in your system.

Pack your hospital bag – You will need to stay in the hospital only one night, so pack whatever you need to make yourself both comfortable and entertained.

Prepare your support group – After your surgery, you will need to have friends and family lined up to prepare and bring you your meals, pick up your prescription medications, help you with minor grooming, etc. They will need to be educated as to what your surgery entailed and what your limitations will be and for how long. Get people committed in helping you during certain days and times to do specific chores, etc., before surgery day.

Get your insurance or money lined up ahead of time – Refer to the insurance information under the steps given in this book and/or review the cost in the FAQ section above.

Get caught up with household chores, even pre-making your protein drinks – After your surgery, you won't want to or be able to do a lot of the things that you normally do for a while, so get ahead of the laundry, the housekeeping, the grocery shopping, clothes shopping, and anything else that you normally do that can be done ahead of time.

While you will (hopefully) have some helpers lined up, it would be helpful to everybody, including yourself, if you had most of the work done ahead of time and utilize your volunteers for things that you can't do ahead of time and would need help with right after surgery.

You will want a lot of smoothies and shakes because they pack a lot of protein in a small amount. You will likely be able to get around in the kitchen at this point, but you won't feel like doing projects, and smoothies and shakes call for fresh ingredients.

Fresh ingredients don't stay fresh for long, and you likely won't feel like driving, shopping and messing around a lot in the kitchen yet. Your helpers most likely will not want to shop for fresh ingredients, follow a recipe, cut and blend things either. That would make them feel imposed upon and regretful they volunteered to help you, so you really need to make smoothies and shakes ahead of time!

Make the smoothies and shakes up, minus the ice the recipes may call for, and pour them into ice cube trays for easy access and measurement into two ounces per cube. You could transfer the frozen smoothie or shake cubes to a container and label the container.

You won't be consuming much of anything for a while. Frozen cubed smoothies and shakes would allow small amounts of your pre-made, frozen smoothies and shakes to be easily accessed. When it is time for you to drink some, you or your helper can take out a couple of cubes and some ice shavings, blend them and pour the drink into your medicine (it has measurements) cup or whatever.

Get the facts – Do your homework and the steps mentioned. Once you have researched everything and talked to the surgeon of your choice, you will feel much more confident when you have your surgery.

Study the proteins – You will need to consume a lot of protein before and after your surgery, so explore and experiment with various sources of protein. Know what they are.

What do I need to take to the hospital?

It is totally up to you what you take to the hospital, but in general, you will want what makes you comfortable and keeps you entertained.

You may want lotion, lip balm, and grooming items. You may want your favorite pillow and/or pillowcase. Things that will make you comfortable clothes-wise may include house slippers for the hospital stay and loose-fitting clothes and slip-on shoes for that trip home.

You may want your electronic gadgets for keeping your family up to date on your progress using social media. You may want to read ebooks or surf the web. You may just want a good physical book or a stack of magazines for your entertainment in addition to the television that you will likely have in your room.

Chapter 6: Your Pre-Operation Diet

If you think that you can binge eat right up until operation day, you are wrong. Not only will you have to have stopped smoking about a month before operation day (to assure better healing), but you will need to have followed a strict diet for a couple of weeks. It is important for you to cooperate with the surgeon by following this diet before the surgery.

Since you are obese, there is a high likelihood that your liver is also full of fat. To access your stomach laparoscopically, the surgeon needs to be able to move your liver to the side. If it is still a fatty liver that he finds during your operation, moving it aside wouldn't make any difference to his inability to access your stomach laparoscopically.

The surgeon will likely cancel the operation or do your operation the open surgery method if you didn't follow instructions to shrink your liver's size through this two-week diet.

If the doctor can do your surgery laparoscopically, he can decrease the risk of complications during your surgery, the surgery will be performed quicker and easier, and you will experience significantly less pain than you would if you force the surgeon to perform the operation in the open surgery method.

The Requirements

Typically, you will be required to change your eating habits as follows:

- Increase protein consumption through lean meats, protein

powders, etc.

- Lower your carbohydrate consumption by avoiding bread, pasta, cereal, rice, etc.

- Eliminate sugar, including candy, desserts, juices, soda, etc.

Two Weeks before your Surgery - Sample Pre-Operation Menu

A sample daily two-week, the pre-operation menu looks like the following:

Breakfast

Protein shake (even just one of the commercially made ones) that does not contain any sort of sugar

Lunch

Lean meat plus vegetables

Dinner

Lean meat plus vegetables

Snacks

Low-carb, healthy options, such as nuts, berries, veggies, small salad with an oil and vinegar dressing

Fluids

Drink lots of fluids that are sugar-free and low in calories

Two Days before Your Surgery – More Limitations

You will need to do the following for the two days before your surgery:

- Omit carbonated beverages

- Omit caffeine

- Go on a diet of clear liquids. Clear food consists of things like broth, sugar-free popsicles, sugar-free Jell-O, and water. You may get one protein shake on each day, but maybe not. You really do need to keep off of sugar during these two days. Follow your surgeon's instructions.

Chapter 7: Your Diet on Surgery Day and Beyond

If you think you can cheat on your diet now, you are wrong! You cannot cheat on your diet after your surgery or you will suffer. Your pre-op diet was for the purpose of reducing risk *during* your surgery. Your post-op diet (the first four weeks after surgery) will be for the purpose of reducing the risk of *post-op complications*.

Your surgeon is not being overly cautious when he tells you to continue to consume clear liquids. It is important that you continue to follow the prescribed diet very closely.

If you cheat on your diet, you may cause a very serious gastric leak, where food gets through the staple line, out of your digestive system and into your abdominal area. If that happens early, the surgeon will get back in there and flush you out. If that happens later, it will progress to an infection that can become life-threatening.

Cheating could also cause constipation, diarrhea, or even bowel obstruction. Just don't do it! Stay the course and you will be able to gradually add back foods that you love without creating problems (and possibly another surgery) for yourself.

You will be in pain after your surgery, so it will be normal for you to be irritable during this time and to wonder whether or not you should have had the surgery. But this too will pass!

Surgery Day – Nothing by Mouth

You will probably be thirsty after your operation, but you won't be allowed to drink anything until the day after your operation. The breathing tube that was put down your throat would make drinking unpleasant anyway. Your surgeon may allow mouth swabs or an occasional cup of ice.

Day One – Drink Test and Discharge Day

A radiologist will give you a swallow test that will test for major leaks in your stomach area before you will be allowed by the surgeon to have water to drink. You should only have a small amount of anything on this day.

No carbonated drinks or drinks with caffeine will be allowed on this day. Caffeine creates a diuretic effect, which is a major reason patients who cheat and drink something with caffeine are readmitted for dehydration!

Don't accept drinks or food from well-meaning family or friends that are off of the list of allowed drinks or food. Follow the doctor's orders. There is a good reason for not consuming whatever he tells you not to consume!

You will likely just be thirsty on this day, but if you do want something other than water, your choices will be as follows:

- Sugar-free gelatin
- Strained cream soup
- Milk
- Unsweetened juice
- Broth

Days Two and Three – On Your Own

Your spouse may be back at work. You will likely need to get whatever you consume on your own unless you have children or unemployed friends lined up to help you after you get home.

What you are allowed to eat on these two days is up to your surgeon. You may still be on the liquid diet for the remainder of the week. Alternatively, you may be allowed to advance to pureed food at some point during your first week following surgery.

If you can have pureed food, it cannot have lumps in it. The food allowed will likely include the following items:

- Soft fruit
- Yogurt
- Fish
- Beans
- Lean ground meat

Liquids allowed will likely include the following:

- Broth
- Juice
- Fat-free milk
- Water

Your body is used to getting a lot of its fluids from food, but it won't get all that it needs from food now. You need to drink a lot of fluids from now on. Check your sugar levels if you are diabetic. Your diabetes meds have likely been reduced now as part of the discharge plan.

Week One – Clear Liquids Only

As previously stated, you won't likely have much desire to eat food right after you have your surgery because the hunger hormone (ghrelin) won't exist within you. That is because the area of the stomach where most of that hormone was manufactured has been removed. You may or may not be off of the clear liquid diet by days two and three.

You cannot have caffeine, sugar, sweet beverages or carbonated beverages at this stage, so your clear-liquid options that you can consume during this early time period consisting of the following:

- Sugar-free drinks (flat or otherwise has no carbonation)
- Sugar-free popsicles
- Decaffeinated coffee
- Decaffeinated tea
- Jell-O
- Broth
- Water

Week Two – Liquid Diet with Protein

You may actually be a little hungry by now, but it will likely be a week that involves tasty protein shakes. Yum! Hopefully, you pre-made, tested, tweaked, and froze a bunch of different flavors of shakes and smoothies before your surgery. Hopefully, the family has stayed out of them too!

Eat whatever the surgeon tells you to eat, but your diet will likely include the following choices:

- Protein powder mixed with a clear liquid that is sugar-free and non-carbonated
- Cream soups thinned out with water and containing no chunks in it
- Soups with soft noodles
- Sugar-free sorbet
- Sugar-free pudding
- Non-fat yogurt
- Sugar-free and very watery hot oatmeal
- Diluted, no sugar added juice
- Thinned applesauce with no sugar added

Week Three – Soft Pureed Food

This will likely be a tough week for you. You will be able to add some normal food to your diet, though pureed, some of it will likely make you sick.

Some food may taste different to you now. Some food may not be tolerated well after your surgery, such as dairy. If you introduce food one by one, you will be able to identify food that you have trouble with so as to avoid it for a while.

You will also document what each offending food did to you. Did it cause gas, upset your stomach, cause diarrhea? If you premade shakes, know what you put into the shakes so that you can document the ingredients from which one or more may not yet agree with your new digestive system.

Continue to limit sugar and fat. This week you have three goals you need to reach, which are:

- Consume 60 grams of protein every day (more if you are a man).
- Eat your food slowly.
- Introduce new food one at a time, not during the same meal.

During this week, you need to AVOID the following items:

- Fibrous vegetables such as broccoli, celery, asparagus and raw leafy greens
- Starchy foods like pasta, rice, and bread
- Sugar – Note: Even your protein smoothies and shakes can have too much sugar in the form of fructose, so you may need to consume those extra fruity drinks in smaller doses than the other smoothies and shakes during this stage.

Food choices for this week include the following items:

- One protein shake or smoothie per day, which can be blended with yogurt   or non-fat milk or even cottage cheese

- Almond milk in shakes

- Coconut milk in shakes

- Hummus

- Low-fat cottage cheese

- Soft cheeses in limited amount (high in fat)

- Soft (soggy) cereal

- Soft steamed or boiled vegetables

- Ground beef mixed with stock to keep it soft

- Ground chicken mixed with stock to keep it soft

- Soups

- Scrambled eggs (good source of protein)

- Canned tuna mixed with low-fat mayonnaise (good source of protein)

- Canned salmon mixed with low-fat mayonnaise (good source of protein)

- Mashed fruit that has not had sugar added to it. Bananas are great

- Mashed avocados

Week Four – Introduce Real Food

While you do not have to eat pureed food this week, you still need to eat softer versions of the various food options and you need to continue to chew your food well.

Your stomach is still sensitive. You need to AVOID the following food items:

- Sodas
- Sugary drinks
- Candy
- Dessert
- Fried foods
- Nuts
- High-carbohydrate food such as pasta, bread, pizza
- Whole milk
- Whole milk dairy foods

This week's menu can contain food such as the following:

- Protein shakes daily
- Beef and chicken introduced slowly and chewed thoroughly
- Fish of any kind
- Vegetables, soft
- Sweet potatoes
- Mashed potatoes
- Baked potatoes
- Cereal
- Caffeine, a limited amount can be introduced

If your surgeon approves of you having *snacks* between meals, they may include foods such as the following:

- Fresh fruit
- One-quarter of a baked sweet potato
- One-quarter cup of oatmeal
- One hard-boiled egg
- Hummus on rice crackers
- Hummus with boiled baby carrots

Week Five to Month Three

Continue to introduce food one by one and notate how well you take each one. Eating something you don't tolerate well will give you constipation, upset stomach, or diarrhea.

You will still eat things like cooked vegetables, canned or soft fruit, ground meat and finely diced meat. Do NOT eat much in the way of solid, hard food yet. You must wait until the doctor clears you for those kinds of foods.

Guidelines

- Eat three meals daily, still concentrating on protein intake.
- Drink lots of fluids throughout every day, but stop drinking 30 minutes before each meal.
- Try not to snack unless you have something nutritious, such as fruit, veggies or maybe a few nuts.
- Remember to take your vitamins.
- Make sure you get around 60 grams of protein (get a little more if you are a man), drinking a protein shake every day

in addition to the small amount of food you are eating.

- Make a habit of doing some sort of exercise every day.

- As always, avoid sodas, although you can have a little bit of caffeine (tea, coffee) now.

- Be prepared for bad days so that you can cope.

- Find yourself an accountability partner in a support group or somewhere that you can call.

Month Three to Month Six and Beyond

You should have lost a very noticeable amount of weight by now and are very glad you had the surgery.

Your surgeon will likely approve you for solid foods now. You will feel full very fast now when you eat them. Chew them well. Eat slowly.

You need to take it slowly because crunchy and/or spicy food may be difficult to tolerate at first. As before, you need to introduce one solid food at a time and see how well your system handles it. Document any problems, as always.

You should have a dietician that you meet with regularly by now. They will help you strategize blending your diet with those of your family's and give you grocery shopping tips and tips for getting through holiday meals, etc.

General Tips

To help you in your journey, here are six useful tips:

- Choose foods that contain a lot of nutrients. For example, fish and fruit contain lots of nutrients, but bread does not have much value.

- Don't drink your calories. Calorie-filled drinks usually contain a lot of sugar and they don't fill you up.

- Create a plan to deal with emotional days when you will be tempted to use food to comfort yourself with.

- Take your time eating your food, chewing everything very thoroughly.

- When you eat out, eat half a portion size. You may be able to split a meal with somebody else who then orders a side dish or two to complete their meal. Alternatively, you could get a box and take half of your meal home with you or see whether or not the restaurant would give you a discount for ordering half a meal.

- Buy yourself a reusable 64-ounce bottle that you can carry with you. Fill it with water and drink all of the water every day, remembering to not drink fluids with meals.

  The reason you should not drink with your meals is that your stomach doesn't hold nearly as much as it did before your surgery, so you need to utilize the space for meals. You also don't want to run the risk of stretching out your stomach pouch. It is possible to stretch it out, accommodating more food, which defeats the purpose of getting the pouch size cut via the sleeve gastrectomy.

Chapter 8: Vitamins and Minerals

Whatever type of gastric surgery you have had, you will need to take vitamins and supplements for the rest of your life. Bypass patients need the most, followed by sleeve patients and then lab band patients.

Even people who have not had gastric surgery should take vitamins and supplements because our food is lacking the nutrition that it used to have. Additionally, people seldom make good food choices.

None of us are getting the nutrition we need in the United States unless we take vitamins and supplements. But for the gastric patient, it is no longer physically possible to take in sufficient nutrients just from food, even if the patient ate only quality food.

A gastric sleeve patient will typically need to take a multivitamin and minerals, iron, calcium citrate, vitamin B12, and protein supplements, although taking more vitamins would be even better. Let's look at each one of these supplements.

Multivitamin and minerals

You will need a chewable multivitamin the first month following your surgery, possibly taking one in the morning and one at night. Bariatric Advantage and Bariatric Fusion are good ones for bariatric patients. Centrum Adult Daily Chewable is an option for the non-bariatric consumer, and it can be found at common local pharmacies such as Walgreens.

Iron

Your surgeon may recommend that you take iron. If he does, he'll tell you to take it on an empty stomach. Do not buy the typical ferrous sulfate because your body will not absorb it after your surgery. What you need is Ferrous Fumarate 29mg. Do not take it when you take your Calcium Citrate, however.

Calcium Citrate

You will start to take this supplement one month after your surgery. You can get it in chewable form or in liquid form. Take this supplement three times daily for a total of between 1500 and 2000 mg. Spread your doses apart by at least one hour in between doses.

As stated in the iron paragraph above, you should not take Calcium Citrate at the same time that you take the iron. In fact, you need to separate taking the Calcium Citrate from when you take both your multivitamin and iron supplements by at least two hours.

Vitamin B12

You typically take this vitamin one time per week at a dosage of between 5000 and 7500 mg. You can get it sublingually (under your tongue), by injection, or by nasal spray. Do not take this in pill form after your surgery.

Protein supplements

You need to have at least 60 mg of protein daily. In supplement form, surgeons prefer that you buy a bariatric-specific protein supplement, such as Bariatric Advantage, Unjury, or Bariatric Fusion, instead of the kind you find at common retailers.

Of course, you will use a lot of protein powder in smoothies and shakes that you make.

There are also a few commercially-made brands that are low enough in sugar to suffice, although you really need to stay away from any with sugar if you can help it. They are as follows:

- MET-Rx Protein Plus – This drink delivers 51 grams of protein and only two grams of sugar within each 260-calorie drink.

- Nature's Best Zero Carb Isopure – This drink delivers up to 40 grams of protein and no carbs within each 160-calorie drink.

- CytoSport Monster Milk – This drink delivers 45 grams of protein and **no sugar** within each drink. It also contains five grams of dietary fiber in every drink.

- Muscle Milk Pro – This drink delivers 40 grams of protein and two grams of sugar in each lactose-free and gluten-free drink. This brand can be found more easily than the others can, and can even be found in gas stations and convenience stores.

- Shakeology – This drink delivers 17 grams of protein and six grams of sugar in each drink, which makes it not the best choice. However, it does give you the added benefit of 70 vitamins, minerals, probiotics, prebiotics, fiber, digestive enzymes, antioxidants, and phytonutrients.

- Pure Protein Shakes – This drink delivers between 23 and 35 grams of protein, depending on the size and flavor, in each drink while including just one gram of sugar and no aspartame. Each drink also gives you three grams of fiber, some calcium, and other benefits.

Chapter 9: Stomach Stretching after Surgery

Besides getting rid of most of the hunger hormone, the other purpose of the surgery is to shrink the stomach size so as to feel full faster. Whether or not the stomach could stretch out, enabling the weight to come back on, is one of the top questions that people ask about gastric sleeve surgery. After all, a person goes through money, pain, trouble and a small risk of complications for the purpose of losing weight and keeping the weight off.

It is possible to stretch the smaller stomach out, but whether or not the stomach stretches back out and the weight returns is up to the patient. The surgery makes the stomach smaller and gets rid of much of the hunger hormones, so the patient is given a good advantage over other people when it comes to keeping the weight off.

This advantage should enable success for the remainder of the patient's life, however, it is possible to mess this up. The patient must actively keep their stomach small.

The other factor affecting the weight gain part of the equation, of course, is whether or not the patient also maintains the new diet and exercise lifestyle. Consuming just sugary and fat food, even in a small stomach, will pack the pounds back on. The surgery is a tool, not a quick fix. The patient must work at his weight loss goal for the rest of his or her life.

Know how hunger and fullness signals get messed up.

Let's take a closer look at how the stomach works. The walls of your stomach contain folds of tissue that expand and contract in response to the food that enters and leaves the stomach. When the stomach expands far enough, a signal goes to your brain that tells it you have eaten enough food. Your stomach is full.

Acid starts to break down the food as soon as it enters. The stomach walls contract to push the food on down to your intestines for further digestion of the food.

If you overeat and stretch the walls too often, the stomach tells the brain that it is full later than it should. It also tells the brain that it is hungry when it still contains food. This broken signal system causes you to eat more food on a regular basis, which is what makes losing weight difficult for people in the first place.

Keep yourself on track using several tricks.

An occasional large meal such as one at Thanksgiving, won't mess up the signals, however, habitual overeating will permanently stretch out your stomach and mess up the signals.

Here are some tips for keeping your stomach small after surgery:

- You already limit the sugar in your diet, which is likely hard for you. Give yourself a reward every week, but make the reward a small sweet treat instead of a large meal, even if it would have been a healthy large meal.

- Don't drink when you eat. Drink your fluids one or two hours before or after you eat so that the fluids don't increase the amount of gas in your system or take up stomach space you need for the small amount of food you will eat.

- After an occasional large meal, make sure that your next meal is small and that you don't make those large ones a habit.

- If you stay hungry, eat small amounts of healthy snacks between your small meals. Almonds make a satisfying and healthy snack.

- Get a good recipe book that is geared for gastric sleeve patients.

- Get back on track, even if you overeat for up to a week. Don't get discouraged. If you have ongoing trouble keeping the amount of food you eat under control, call your surgeon.

- Ask for helpful information from people in the online forums. You are anonymous there anyway.

Take control of the portion size when others try to control it.

The restaurants often serve portion sizes that are already enough for two smallish adults. They make more money by doing that. When you eat at a restaurant or in some other situation, such as at somebody's home, where somebody else tries to control your portion size, you must take control of how much food you eat during that meal.

In those restaurant situations, you can take control of your portion size (and save a lot of money over time) the following ways:

- Get a box to take the other half of your meal home to eat later.

- Split the meal with somebody you are eating out with.

- Request a lunch size.

- Order a couple of side dishes or an appetizer instead of a full meal.

At somebody's home, tell the person who is putting food on your plate how much you want.

The bottom line is that you must actively keep your stomach small.

Conclusion

Thank you again for downloading this book!

I hope this book was able to answer many questions that you may have had about the gastric sleeve procedure and that it helped those of you who have not yet had a sleeve gastrectomy to be confident in your choice to have the surgery and to know what to do before and after you have it.

Hopefully, those of you who have already gone through the procedure realize how important it is to not cheat on your diet, and you hopefully also have a good understanding of how to succeed in keeping the weight off once you are out of the danger zone.

If you have not yet had your surgery and you are confident in your decision to have it, the next step is to follow the steps outlined in Chapter Three. The surgeon you choose is an especially important factor in reducing the risk of having complications during and as a result of the surgery.

After your surgery, you need to stay on the diet and follow all of your doctor's instructions because your food choices during the recovery time directly affect the risk factor for having complications that could become life-threatening. That will not the time to cheat!

Going forward after the recovery period, you must fight your urges to eat sweets, fattening food or to overeat. You've been through a lot. Now the hard work begins. It is so worth it, though.

Gastric Sleeve Recipes

Making Bariatric Surgery Recovery Palatable

© **Copyright 2017 by John Carter - All rights reserved.**

The following eBook is reproduced below with the goal of providing information that is as accurate and as reliable as possible. Regardless, purchasing this eBook can be seen as consent to the fact that both the publisher and the author of this book are in no way experts on the topics discussed within, and that any recommendations or suggestions made herein are for entertainment purposes only. Professionals should be consulted as needed before undertaking any of the action endorsed herein.

This declaration is deemed fair and valid by both the American Bar Association and the Committee of Publishers Association and is legally binding throughout the United States.

Furthermore, the transmission, duplication or reproduction of any of the following work, including precise information, will be considered an illegal act, irrespective whether it is done electronically or in print. The legality extends to creating a secondary or tertiary copy of the work or a recorded copy and is only allowed with express written consent of the Publisher. All additional rights are reserved.

The information in the following pages is broadly considered to be a truthful and accurate account of facts, and as such any inattention, use or misuse of the information in question by the reader will render any resulting actions solely under their purview. There are no scenarios in which the publisher or the original author of this work can be in any fashion deemed liable for any hardship or damages that may befall them after undertaking information described herein.

Additionally, the information found on the following pages is intended for informational purposes only and should thus be considered, universal. As befitting its nature, the information presented is without assurance regarding its continued validity or interim quality. Trademarks that mentioned are done without written consent and can in no way be considered an endorsement from the trademark holder.

Bonus:

FREE Report Reveals The Secrets To Lose Weight

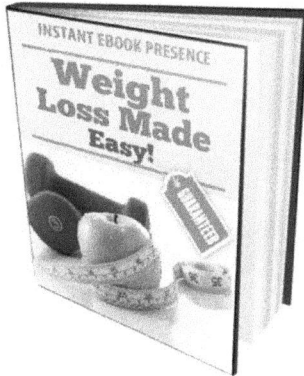

Weight loss doesn't happen from dieting only. Diets are short term solutions to shed extra weight. Diets do not work in the long term because people hate being on a diet (it's ok, you can admit that here). The only long term solution for permanent weight loss is to create new eating habits. This doesn't mean that chocolate will never pass your lips again, but it does mean looking after yourself and watching what you eat...

You can lose weight when you have the right reasons and motivation, and a part of this guide is to help you to find the motivation you need to change your weight...

Go to Get This Guide For FREE

http://www.sportsforsoul.com/weight-loss-2/

Table of Contents

Introduction

I want to thank you and congratulate you for downloading the book, *"Gastric Sleeve Recipes: Making Bariatric Surgery Recovery Palatable."*

After surgery, your diet's ingredient choices will be few, but they will broaden as the weeks go by. Tempted as you may be, you cannot cheat on a bariatric diet or you will suffer some unpleasant consequences. It is, therefore, important for you to enjoy your food as much as possible so that you won't be tempted to cheat on your diet. That is where this little book can help you.

Your first two weeks will consist of just a few liquid choices, so this book contains recipes for weeks three onward. Entire chapters are devoted to week three, week four, week five through month three, and month three onward. Each chapter is divided into recipe choices for meals, side dishes, snacks, desserts, and drinks.

It is important that you get an established amount of protein in your diet every day, which is usually around 60 grams for women and 70 grams for men. In addition to protein-rich food recipes, this book contains many recipes for delicious protein shakes and smoothies. Protein drinks will help you to easily reach the daily protein intake goal that your surgeon will establish for you.

The shakes are so delicious and healthy, they will likely become some of your lifetime favorites! A few fruit drinks are also included in the drink sections.

There are plenty of books on this subject on the market, thanks again for choosing this one! Every effort was made to ensure it is full of as much useful information as possible. Please enjoy!

Chapter 1:
Week Three (Soft Pureed Food) Recipes

After one long week with just **clear, sugar-free liquids** and a week that allowed you to add **thinned cream and/or soft noodle soups, sugar-free pudding, sugar-free sorbet, and non-fat yogurt** to the list, now you can have a few more satisfying foods. However, *the new food items must be pureed.*

Even pureed, we now have enough food ingredients that we can start to put together some tasty food options using simple recipes. This week, you can add the following ingredients, remembering to mash, blend or puree them:

- **Mashed avocado**
- **Mashed fruit, i.e. bananas**
- **Canned salmon**
- **Canned tuna**
- **Scrambled eggs**
- **Soups**
- **Ground chicken with stock**
- **Ground beef with stock**
- **Boiled vegetables**
- **Steamed vegetables**
- **Soggy cereal**
- **Soft cheese, limited amount**
- **Low-fat cottage cheese**
- **Low-fat mayonnaise**
- **Hummus**
- **Coconut milk**
- **Almond milk**
- **Protein shake or smoothie - one per day, blended with yogurt, non-fat milk or cottage cheese**

You need to **AVOID** the following items:
- Sugar
- Starchy foods
- Fibrous vegetables

Goals
- Consume 60 grams of protein every day and about 70 grams if you are a man (or whatever your doctor tells you).
- Eat your food slowly.
- Introduce only one new food from the list above per meal, notating any food intolerances.

Introduce only one of the aforementioned new food items per meal and take notice of whether or not your body reacts to the food. You may get nauseated and vomit or have other reactions, so you don't want to introduce more than one item at a time.

Some recipes do combine several ingredients, so if one meal upsets your system, you may want to go back to a clear liquid diet for a day and then move on to a different new food.

On a later date, you can divide the components of that offending meal up and try one new ingredient during a meal and then another one the next meal to figure out which ingredient your system wasn't taking (i.e. separate the beef from the guacamole or try beef with no spices). You want to know what to avoid for a while!

Take physical notes of what the offending food was that you tried to add, how your body reacted to it, etc.

To get the required amount of protein daily, you'll want to take advantage of shakes and smoothies because the protein powder in them give you a lot of protein per sip!

Meal Recipes

Beef with Avocado
Serving: 1
Prep and Cooking Time: 00:40:00

What to Use

- Ground beef chuck (.5 pound, cooked and grease drained off)
- Beef stock
- Avocado (one, mashed)
- Powdered Onion
- Mild Mexican spices
- Salt (pinch)
- Black pepper (pinch)
- Lemon (to taste, optional)
- Soft cheese (.125 cup of optional soft cheese)

What to Do

- Fry up the hamburger. Drain all grease off of it.
- Put cooked beef in blender with enough beef stock to give it a soft, pureed consistency.
- Add mild spices to taste, if desired.
- Turn out hamburger mixture into a small bowl.
- Peel and seed the avocado
- Blend the avocado until creamy in blender. Add lemon and/or onion powder to avocado to taste.
- Take out anything hard.
- Coat the avocado mixture over the hamburger mixture.

Tuna with Low-Fat Mayonnaise

Servings: 1-2
Prep Time: 00:10:00

What to Use

- Tuna (1 large can)
- Onion (.25 onion, boiled or steamed)
- Salt (to taste)
- Pepper (to taste)
- Low-fat mayonnaise (to taste)

What to Do

- Boil or steam the onion
- Blend onion until cut into small pieces.
- Add tuna and blend until there are no chunks.
- Add the remaining ingredients and blend, adding ingredients until it suits   your taste.
- Chill and serve alone as a cold salad, or warm it up if preferred warm.

Chicken with Broth

Serving: 1
Prep and Cooking Time: 00:20:00

What to Use

- Chicken (1 breast, cooked and pureed)
- Chicken broth (.25 cup)
- Salt (pinch)
- Black pepper (pinch)

What to Do

- Cook the chicken breast.
- Cut up the chicken breast into a few large cubes and put into blender.
- Pulse the chicken breast in the blender a few times.
- Add the chicken stock to the chicken and blend until well pureed.
- Season to flavor

Tuna with Cheese

Serving: 1
Prep Time: 00:10:00

What to Use

- Tuna (one 5-ounce can, mashed or pureed)
- Low-fat cheese (to taste)

What to Do

- Puree tuna with low-fat cheese.
- Heat up and enjoy.

Side Dish Recipes

Cream of Avocado Soup

Servings: 2

Prep and Cooking Time: 00:15:00

What to Use

- Cream of Chicken soup (2 cups of prepared, liquified soup)
- Avocado (one soft, pared and seeded)
- Salt
- Black pepper

What to Do

- Peel and seed the avocado.
- Blend avocado in blender until creamy.
- Prepare cream of chicken soup with water as directed.
- Pour soup into blender and add seasonings to taste.
- Blend until smooth.
- Strain out anything hard.
- Heat it up and serve.

Cooked Carrots with Hummus
Several Servings
Prep and Cooking Time: 00:15:00

What to Use

- Garbanzo beans (2 cups, canned, drained)
- Garlic (2 cloves, halved)
- Lemon juice (.25 cup)
- Tahini (.33 cup)
- Salt (One tsp)
- Olive oil (One tbsp)
- Paprika (pinch)
- Carrots (several, as desired)

What to Do

- Slice, steam and mash the carrots. Put carrots into several serving bowls.
- Blend the first five ingredients together in a blender to make the hummus.
- Put the hummus.
- Trickle olive oil.
- Strew with paprika (After you are further along in your bariatric diet, you can also sprinkle chopped, fresh parsley on top).

Buttery Mixed Vegetables

Servings: 2
Prep and Cooking Time: 00:10:00

What to Use

- Mixed vegetables (1 can, drained)
- Butter Buds
- Salt
- Black pepper

What to Do

- Open can of vegetables. Drain off juices.
- Add salt, pepper and Butter Buds.
- Heat over stove or in microwave oven.
- Dish up and serve.

Snack Recipes

Protein-Rich Yogurt

Serving: 1
Prep Time: 00:10:00

What to Use

- Low-fat, sugar-free yogurt (single serving, flavor of your choice)
- Protein powder (1-2 scoops, flavor of your choice)

What to Do

- Mix the protein powder with the yogurt.
- Top with any sugar-free, low-fat topping.

Pureed Deviled Eggs

Servings: 3-6
Prep and Cooking Time: 00:20:00

What to Use

- Eggs (6 hard boiled, pureed)
- Dry mustard (.5 teaspoon)
- Salt (.5 teaspoon)
- Black pepper (.25 teaspoon)
- Low-fat mayonnaise (3 tablespoons)

What to Do

- Boil the eggs.
- Blend/puree the cooked eggs in blender.
- Add spices and low-fat mayonnaise. Makes enough for several breakfasts and/or snacks.

Dessert Recipes

Cheesecake Protein Pudding

Servings: 2
Calories: 220.3
Prep and Cooking Time: 00:15:00

What to Use

- Dymatize ISO 100 Gourmet Vanilla Protein Powder by Daymonm2 (2-serving)
- Almond Breeze Almond Milk, unsweetened (4 ounces)
- Non-fat cottage cheese (1 cup, not packed, drained)

What to Do

- Drain liquid from the cottage cheese.
- Put all ingredients into your Magic Bullet or blender. Blend.
- Chill.

Jell-O with Bananas

Servings: 6
Prep and Cooking Time: 00:15:00

What to Use

- Jell-O (1 small package, unsweetened in any flavor)
- Banana (1 banana, mashed)
- Sugar-free whipped topping (to taste)

What to Do

- Mix Jell-O powder with water and put into pan as directed on the package.
- Mash the banana and put it into the Jell-O.
- Chill as usual.
- Serve with sugar-free whipped topping.

Flavored Cottage Cheese

Servings: 2
Prep Time: 00:15:00

What to Use

- Low-fat cottage cheese (16 ounces)
- Sugar-free Jell-O powder (1 small envelope)

What to Do

- Drain the cottage cheese.
- Put cottage cheese into the blender or into a mixing bowl.
- Pour the dry Jell-O powder in with the cottage cheese.
- Blend together.

Fruit with Whipped Cream

Serving: 1
Prep Time: 00:10:00

What to Use

- Fruit (.5 cup, soft fruit of your choice, in natural juices)
- Cool Whip Lite (to taste)

What to Do

- Mash or puree fruit.
- Top with sugar-free Cool Whip

Sugar-Free Chocolate Mousse

Servings: 3
Prep Time: 00:10:00

What to Use

- Raw cacao powder (2 tablespoons)
- Avocado (1 ripe)
- Coconut milk (1 small can)

What to Do

- Blend in blender until smooth.
- Pour into 3 small serving cups.
- Chill

Drink Recipes

Peach Cobbler Shake

Servings: 3
Prep Time: 00:10:00

What to Use

- Almond milk (.5 cup, unsweetened)
- Peaches (.5 cup, sliced, fresh or frozen)
- Vanilla protein powder (1 scoop)
- Cinnamon (dash)
- Ice (4-5 cubes)

What to Do

- Blend all ingredients

Pumpkin Pie Shake

Servings: 3
Prep Time: 00:10:00

What to Use

- Banana (.33 banana, frozen)
- Almond milk (.5 cup, unsweetened)
- Pumpkin puree (.25 cup)
- Pumpkin pie spice (to taste)
- Vanilla protein powder (1 scoop)

What to Do

- Blend all ingredients

Milk Shake

Servings: 2
Prep Time: 00:15:00

What to Use

- Skim or non-dairy milk (1 cup)
- Protein powder (1-2 scoops, any flavor)
- Ice (6 cubes, could be frozen skim or non-dairy milk)

What to Do

- Blend all ingredients

Chocolaty Banana Protein Shake

Servings: 2
Prep Time: 00:10:00

What to Use

- Water or nonfat milk (.5 cup)
- Banana (one, frozen)
- Chocolate protein powder (1 scoop)
- Ice (1 cup, cubes)

What to Do

- Blend all ingredients

Cookies and Cream Protein Shake

Servings: 2
Prep Time: 00:10:00

What to Use

- Skim milk (.5 cup)
- Cookies and cream protein (1 scoop)
- Vanilla extract (.5 teaspoon)
- Cool Whip Lite (One tbsp)
- Ice (1 cup, cubes)

What to Do

- Blend all ingredients

Angel Food Heaven

Servings: 2
Prep Time: 00:10:00

What to Use

- Almond milk (1 cup, unsweetened)
- Coconut extract (.5 teaspoon)
- Vanilla extract (.5 teaspoon)
- Vanilla protein powder (1 scoop)
- Ice (5-6 cubes)

What to Do

- Blend all ingredients

Pumpkin Protein Shake

Servings: 2
Prep Time: 00:10:00

What to Use

- Pumpkin puree (.25 cup)
- Skim or soy milk (1 cup)
- Pumpkin spice (.25 teaspoon), or cinnamon (.25 teaspoon), or cloves (.125 teaspoon), or ginger (.125 teaspoon)
- Vanilla protein powder (1 scoop)
- Cool Whip Lite (.25 cup)
- Splenda (2 tablespoons, granular)
- Ice (1 cup, cubes)

What to Do

- Blend all except for the ice.
- Add ice one cube at a time until it reaches the desired consistency.
- Pour into glass.
- Top with Cool Whip too if desired.

Banana Protein Shake
Serving: 1
Prep Time: 00:10:00

What to Use

- Skim milk (1 cup)
- Banana (one 1-inch chunk)
- Vanilla protein powder (1 scoop)
- Vanilla (.5 teaspoon)
- Nutmeg (.125 teaspoon)

What to Do

- Blend and pour into a glass.

Orange Shake
Serving: 1
Protein: 28 grams
Prep Time: 00:10:00

What to Use

- Skim milk (8 ounces), or orange juice (4 ounces) plus skim milk (4 ounces), or yogurt (4 ounces) plus skim milk (4 ounces)
- Vanilla whey protein powder (1 scoop)
- Sunrise Orange Crystal Light powder (1 scoop, sugar-free)

What to Do

- Blend and pour into a glass.

Icy Apple Pie Refresher

Servings: 2
Prep Time: 00:10:00

What to Use

- Water (.75 cup)
- Applesauce (.5 cup, no sugar added)
- HDT 5+1 vanilla protein powder (1.5 scoops)
- Splenda (2 packets)
- Cinnamon (.5 teaspoon)
- Nutmeg (.25 teaspoon)
- Ice (8-10 cubes)

What to Do

- Blend all except for the ice.
- Add ice one cube at a time until it reaches the desired consistency.

Lemon-Ginger Green Juice

Servings: 4
Prep Time: 00:30:00

What to Use

- Cucumber (1 medium, sliced)
- Celery (8 stalks, separated and washed)
- Ginger (.5-inch knob, fresh, peeled)
- Red pepper (one, sliced)
- Apple (1 Fuji or Honeycrisp, sliced)
- Lemon (skin removed)
- Lime (skin removed)

What to Do

- Prep all ingredients that need preparing (washing, cutting, skin removing).
- Use a juice machine, feeding soft pieces and hard pieces alternately.
- Refrigerate.

Romaine Green Juice

Servings: 2
Prep Time: 00:30:00

What to Use

- Romaine lettuce (1 head, leaves separated and washed)
- Carrots (10 medium carrots)
- Parsley (1 bunch)
- Cucumbers (2 medium)
- Celery (8 stalks, separated and washed)
- Ginger (one 1-inch knob, fresh)
- Lemon (1 medium, skin removed)
- Lime (1 small, skin removed)

What to Do

- Prep all ingredients that need preparing (washing, cutting, skin removing) the night before the morning you want to drink it. Store in air-tight container and chill overnight.
- Juice the veggies in juice machine and drink immediately. Store leftover juice in airtight container in refrigerator.

Tasty Beet Juice

Servings: 2
Prep Time: 00:30:00

What to Use

- Beet (1 large, fresh)
- Cucumbers (2 medium, preferably organic)
- Carrots (2 large)
- Lemon (one, skin cut off)
- Lime (one, skin cut off)
- Flat-leaf parsley (1 small bunch)
- Ginger (1.5-inch piece, fresh, skin cut off)

What to Do

- Prep all ingredients that need preparing (washing, cutting, skin removing) the night before the morning you want to drink it. Store in airtight container and chill overnight.
- Juice the veggies in juice machine and drink immediately. Store leftover juice in airtight container in refrigerator.

Celery Zinger Juice

Servings: 2
Prep Time: 00:30:00

What to Use

- Celery (1 head, stalk separated, washed, leaf parts removed, chopped into three or four sections per stalk)
- Flat-leaf parsley (1 small bunch)
- Limes (2 small, skins cut off)
- Red or green apple (1 small)
- Cucumber (1 large, washed)
- Ginger (1.5-inch, fresh)

What to Do

- Prep all ingredients that need preparing (washing, cutting, skin removing) the night before the morning you want to drink it. Store in airtight container and chill overnight.
- Juice the veggies in juice machine and drink immediately. Store leftover juice in airtight container in refrigerator.

Spiced Apple Cider

Servings: 4-8
Prep Time: 00:30:00

What to Use

- Apple cider (2 quarts, unsweetened)
- Allspice (One tsp)
- Cinnamon stick (one stick)
- Whole cloves (several)
- Lemon juice (.25 cup, optional)
- Orange juice (2 tablespoons, optional)
- Sugar-free sweetener (to taste, optional)

What to Do

- Simmer the cider, allspice, cinnamon and cloves over stove for 15 mins.
- Strain.
- Add lemon juice, orange juice, and/or sweetener just before serving, if desired.

Citrus Juice with Mint

Servings: 1
Prep Time: 00:10:00

What to Use

- Orange juice (.5 cup)
- Lemon juice (.5 cup)
- Mint sprig (1 sprig)

What to Do

- Pour the juices into glass.
- Crush sprig of mint and put into the juice.
- Chill for two hours before drinking.

Mango in the Morning

Servings: 1
Prep Time: 00:10:00

What to Use

- Water (2 ounces)
- Lime (.5 lime, fresh-squeezed)
- Mango (one)
- Ginger (small piece, fresh)
- Vanilla or almond extract (One tsp)
- ProScore Vanilla (2 scoops)
- Ice (7-8 cubes)

What to Do

- Blend everything except the protein and ice.
- Add and blend ice one cube at a time until it reaches the desired consistency.

Yummy Peach and Strawberry Refresher

Servings: 1
Prep Time: 00:10:00

What to Use

- Water (.25 - .5 cup)
- Strawberries (3 large berries, frozen)
- Peaches (3 slices) or banana (.5 banana)
- Splenda (1 packet)
- Vanilla protein powder (1 scoop)

What to Do

- Blend and serve.

Chapter 2: Week Four
(Introducing Real Food) Recipes

You are not locked into pureed food this week, but you need to eat soft versions of the newly-introduced food options and to chew everything well.

You've got a sensitive stomach. **AVOID** the following items:

- Whole milk dairy foods
- Whole milk
- Fried food
- Nuts
- Pasta, bread, pizza and other high-carbohydrate food
- Candy
- Desserts containing sugar, fat, etc.
- Sugary drinks
- Sodas

This week you can add the following items, prepared normally:

- **Sweet potatoes**
- **Mashed potatoes**
- **Baked potatoes**
- **Cereal**
- **Fish (any kind)**
- **Chicken**
- **Beef**
- **Caffeine – limited amount**

Snacks your surgeon may let you have now include:

- **Hummus on rice crackers**
- **One-quarter cup of oatmeal**
- **Fresh fruit**
- **One hard-boiled egg**

Goals

- Consume 60 grams of protein every day and a little more if you are a man.
- Eat your food slowly.
- Re-introduce new food from last week's list that you did not tolerate or add items from the list above per meal, notating any food intolerances.

As before, take notice of whether or not your body reacts to new food. You may get nauseated and vomit or have other reactions. Introduce one new meal, side, etc., at a time so that you can narrow down what food or ingredient you are reacting to.

Take physical notes of what the offending food was that you tried to add, how your body reacted to it, etc. Try it again at a later time. Move on to a different new food from the list on your next meal.

To get the required amount of protein daily, you'll want to take advantage of shakes and smoothies because the protein powder in them give you a lot of protein per sip!

Meal Recipes

Curried Coconut Chicken

Servings: 4
Prep and Cooking Time: 01:10:00

What to Use
- Chicken breast halves (2 pounds, boneless, skinless, cut into chunks)
- Onion (.5 onion, thinly sliced)
- Garlic (2 cloves, crushed)
- Stewed, diced tomatoes (one 14.5-ounce can)
- Vegetable oil (1.5 tablespoons)
- Curry powder (2 tablespoons)
- Coriander (.5 teaspoon, crushed)
- Salt and pepper (One tsp)
- Coconut milk (one 14-ounce can)
- Tomato sauce (one 8-ounce can)
- Sweetener (equal to 3 tablespoons sugar)

What to Do
- Slice the onion into thin slices. Set aside.
- Crush the garlic. Set aside.
- Cut the chicken into chunks. Flavor with pepper and salt. Set aside.
- Toss the curry powder and coriander in the skillet for 2 mins. Follow onions and the crushed garlic.
- Put the chicken chunks into the skillet. Toss chicken to coat all sides with the oil for 10 mins.
- Pour in tomato sauce, tomatoes, coconut milk and sugar. Stir together, cover and simmer. Stir occasionally while it simmers for 30 – 40 mins.

Baked Cod Fish

Servings: 1
Prep and Cooking Time: 01:10:00

What to Use

- Cod fish (one, scaled and deboned; could use other lean fish)
- Olive oil
- Butter Buds
- Salt (pinch)
- Black pepper (pinch)
- Lemon pepper (optional)

What to Do

- Place wax paper in shallow baking dish.
- Grease/oil paper with healthy olive oil.
- Place scaled and deboned fish into paper-lined dish.
- Coat a thin layer of olive oil on top of fish.
- Season to flavor
- Bake at 400 degrees in medium-hot oven 20 mins for fillets, 30 mins for steaks, or for 10 mins per pound for a whole fish.
- Serve with sprinkle of lemon pepper if desired.

Baked Hash

Servings: 1
Prep and Cooking Time: 00:50:00

What to Use

- Roast beef (.5 cup, chopped, cooked)
- Potato (.5 cup, diced, cooked)
- Minced onion
- Pimiento (optional)
- Bell pepper (optional)
- Salt
- Black pepper
- Brown gravy
- Olive oil (enough to grease pan)

What to Do

- Dice the potatoes. Bake or otherwise cook the potatoes.
- Adjust oven heat oven to 350 degrees Fahrenheit.
- Grease bottom of a baking dish with olive oil.
- Finely chop the roast, taking off the fat as you go.
- In a bowl, mix the chopped roast, potatoes, minced onion, other desired vegetables, seasonings and brown gravy.
- Transfer to the greased baking dish. Bake for 30 mins.

Hamburger Patty with Minced Garlic and Worcestershire Sauce

Servings: 1
Prep and Cooking Time: 00:15:00

What to Use

- Lean hamburger (enough for one hamburger patty)
- Worcestershire sauce (to taste)
- Garlic (to taste, minced)
- Salt (to taste)
- Black pepper (to taste)

What to Do

- Form patty with your hands.
- Fry patty in a skillet, turning over so as to cook both sides and to not burn one side. A grill would be better for draining fat away as it cooks.
- When you are almost done, add salt and pepper, Worcestershire and minced garlic. Turn patty a time or two. You may have to reapply ingredients.
- Eat without a bun. Eat with grilled or baked veggies on the side.

Simple Breakfast Oatmeal

Servings: 1
Prep and Cooking Time: 00:10:00

What to Use

- Oats (.25 cup, dry)
- Water (to taste)
- Sugar-free brown sugar or sweetener (to taste)
- Fruit (.125 cup, soft, diced, optional)

What to Do

- Add water to oatmeal and boil or microwave until done.
- Add sweetening agent and stir.

Side Dish Recipes

Cooked Vegetables with Cheese Sauce

Servings: 1
Prep and Cooking Time: 00:15:00

What to Use

- Vegetables (.5 cup, cooked)
- Low-fat American cheese (1 slice)

What to Do

- Cook or heat up soft vegetable of your choice.
- Put onto plate.
- Top with cheese, as is, and heated up, or melt first with low-fat milk to make a cheese sauce.

Candied Sweet Potatoes

Servings: 1
Prep and Cooking Time: 00:15:00

What to Use

- Sweet potato (one, cooked and mashed)
- Low-fat milk (to taste)
- Salt (pinch)
- Butter Buds (to taste)
- Sugar-free brown sugar (to taste, for candied touch)

What to Do

- Peel potatoes. Dice into large chunks.
- Boil potatoes until soft.
- Mash potatoes until smooth, adding low-fat milk to thin out.
- Season with Butter Buds, salt, and sugar-free brown sugar to taste.

Baked Potato

Servings: 1
Prep and Cooking Time: 00:15:00

What to Use

- Russet potato (one)
- Low-fat sour cream (.25 cup or to taste)
- American cheese (.25 cup or to taste)
- Butter Buds (to taste)
- Salt (pinch)
- Black Pepper (pinch)

What to Do

- Set the oven to 425 degrees Fahrenheit.
- Wrap potato in aluminum foil. Stab three or four times through foil and into the potato.
- Bake the potato in oven about an hour.
- Take out of the oven and unwrap. Cut in half.
- Add Butter Buds, salt and pepper.
- Add the cheese. If the spud is still hot, the cheese will melt.
- Add sour cream.

Tasty Real Mashed Potatoes

Servings: 1
Prep and Cooking Time: 00:15:00

What to Use

- White potato (one, cooked and mashed)
- Low-fat milk
- Butter Buds
- Seasonings (pepper and salt)

What to Do

- Peel potatoes. Dice into large chunks.
- Boil potatoes until soft.
- Mash potatoes until smooth, adding low-fat milk to thin out to taste.
- Season with salt, pepper and Butter Buds to taste.

Snack Recipes

Buttery Boiled Egg

Servings: 1
Prep and Cooking Time: 00:15:00

What to Use

- Egg (one, hard boiled)
- Butter Buds (pinch)
- Salt (pinch)
- Black pepper (pinch)

What to Do

- Boil egg. Drain off hot water and replace with cold water. Let egg sit in cold water for a few mins to bring the egg's temperature down.
- Take shell off the egg (a spoon works great).
- Put the egg in a serving bowl and chop it up with a fork.
- Sprinkle Butter Buds, salt and pepper on it to taste.

Egg Salad
Servings: 1
Prep and Cooking Time: 00:15:00

What to Use

- Egg (one, hard boiled)
- Low-fat mayonnaise (to taste)
- Onion flakes (to taste)
- Salt (pinch)
- Black pepper (pinch)

What to Do

- Boil egg. Drain off hot water and replace with cold water. Let egg sit in cold water for a few mins to bring the egg's temperature down.
- Take shell off the egg (a spoon works great).
- Put the egg in a serving bowl and chop it up with a fork.
- Add mayo, onion flakes, Butter Buds, salt and pepper on it to taste.
- Allow it time for the onions flakes to soak up the mayo, possibly in the refrigerator to chill at the same time. Nothing hard can be eaten at this point

Dessert Recipes

Fruit Cup with Whipped Cream

Servings: 1
Prep Time: 00:10:00

What to Use

- Fruit cocktail (one cup or can, unsweetened)
- Sugar-free sweetener (to taste, optional)
- Sugar-free Cool Whip

What to Do

- Mix in sweetener, if desired.
- Dish up the amount of fruit you want.
- Top with whip topping.

Banana Pudding with Banana Slices

Servings: 1

Prep Time: 00:10:00

What to Use

- Sugar-free banana pudding (1 small package, as directed but use low-fat milk)
- Banana (.25 of a banana)
- Sugar-free Cool Whip

What to Do

- Make the pudding using low-fat milk.
- Cut .25 off of banana. Cut slices and put on top in into pudding.
- Top with whip topping.

Death by Chocolate High-Protein Pudding

Servings: 1
Prep Time: 00:10:00
Calories: 118.5

What to Use

- Tofu (.5 package = 7.5 ounces, any variety)
- Cocoa, unsweetened (.33 cup)
- Splenda (.75 cup)
- Cinnamon (to taste)
- Nutmeg (to taste)

What to Do

- Cut the tofu into pieces
- Blend all ingredients together until very smooth.
- Pour into .5-cup containers. Cover and chill 1-2 hours.

Cinnamon Roll Cottage Cheese

Servings: 1
Prep Time: 00:10:00

What to Use

- Low-fat cottage cheese (.5 cup, drained)
- Vanilla extract (to taste)
- Cinnamon (to taste)
- Artificial sweetener (to taste)

What to Do

- Blend and serve.

Drink Recipes

Cherry Vanilla Shake
Servings: 1
Prep Time: 00:10:00

What to Use

- Sugar-free cherry yogurt (.5 cup)
- Cherry extract (to taste)
- Vanilla extract (to taste)
- Vanilla powder (1 scoop)
- Water (a splash)
- Ice (4 cubes)

What to Do

- Blend all except for the ice.
- Add ice one cube at a time until it reaches the desired consistency.

Chocolate-Coconut Shake

Servings: 1
Prep Time: 00:10:00

What to Use

- Coconut milk (2 ounces)
- Chocolate sugar-free pudding (One tsp), or banana sugar-free pudding
- Chocolate protein powder (2 scoops)
- Water (6 ounces, cold)

What to Do

- Shake by hand, very well.

Chocolate Raspberry Shake

Servings: 1
Prep Time: 00:10:00

What to Use
- Water or skim milk (8 ounces)
- ProScore 100 chocolate (2 scoops)
- Sugar-free raspberry syrup (to taste)

What to Do
- Blend, pour into a glass and enjoy!

Old Fashioned Vanilla Ice Cream Shake

Servings: 1
Prep Time: 00:10:00

What to Use

- Vitamite (5 ounces)
- DaVinci's Sugar-Free Vanilla Syrup (1 capful)
- GNC 100% Whey Vanilla Protein Powder (1.5 scoop)
- Splenda (4-5 packets)
- Ice (lots of cubes)

What to Do

- Blend all together except for the protein powder and the ice.
- Add the protein powder and briefly blend.
- Add and blend ice one cube at a time until you reach the desired consistency.

Chocolate-Orange Refresher

Servings: 1
Prep Time: 00:10:00

What to Use

- Water (8 ounces)
- ProScore 100 chocolate (1.5 scoops)
- OrangeSicle protein powder (.5 scoop)

What to Do

- Blend, pour into a glass and enjoy!

Delicious Protein Smoothie

Servings: 1
Prep Time: 00:10:00

What to Use
- Sunrise Orange Crystal Light (6-8 ounces)
- Vanilla protein powder (1 scoop)
- Raspberries (to taste, frozen)
- Cool Whip (sugar-free, optional)
- Ice (3 cubes)

What to Do
- Make the Crystal Light. Set aside all but 6-8 ounces of it.
- Blend in the frozen raspberries to taste.
- Add ice cubes one at a time and blend.
- Add the protein last, blending just a few seconds so it won't foam.
- Top with sugar-free Cool Whip if desired.

Chocolate Vanilla Swirl
Servings: 1
Prep Time: 00:10:00

What to Use
- Vanilla protein powder (.5 scoop)
- Chocolate protein powder (.5 scoop)
- Vitamite (a splash)
- Water (a splash)
- Ice (cubes, to taste)

What to Do
- Blend all ingredients

Double Chocolate Fudge Shake
Servings: 1
Prep Time: 00:10:00

What to Use
- Chocolate protein powder (1 scoop)
- Sugar-free hot cocoa mix (1 packet)
- Skim milk (.5 cup)
- Ice (4 cubes)

What to Do
- Blend all ingredients except for ice.
- Add and blend ice cubes one at a time until you reach the desired consistency.

Chapter 3: Week Five to Month Three

During this time, you will continue to introduce different food back into your diet one meal at a time to see how your system tolerates it. Food not tolerated will make you nauseated, constipated and/or have diarrhea.

You will continue to drink lots (64 ounces) of fluid daily and stop drinking fluid 30 mins before you eat.

You will continue to eat **ground meat, finely diced meat, cooked vegetables, canned fruit and soft fresh fruit, among other items mentioned in previous chapters**. Continue to chew them well and to eat slowly. As for hard food, you must **wait until your doctor clears you to eat hard food. This will likely be near the end of this period.**

Try to eat three meals daily and only snack on nutritious food. Continue to concentrate on taking in a lot of protein (60 grams for a female, 70 or so for a male), drinking one shake per day to achieve it. **A little bit of caffeine in the form of tea or coffee is okay** now, but skip the sodas.

Remember to take your vitamins and to get some exercise.

Meal Recipes

Baked Codfish Balls
Servings: 4
Prep and Cooking Time: 00:30:00

What to Use

- Codfish (1 cup, soaked and shredded)
- Potatoes (2 cups, diced)
- Egg (One, beaten)
- Salt (pinch)
- Black pepper (pinch)
- Butter Buds (to taste)

What to Do

- Soak the codfish.
- Shred the codfish.
- Set oven to 350F
- Grease a baking pan with olive oil.
- Beat the eggs.
- Mix the codfish, potatoes, Butter Buds, salt and pepper together with the shredded codfish.
- Form into balls.
- Instead of dipping in flour and frying them, bake them in the preheated oven until done.

Banana Almond Breakfast Oatmeal

Servings: 1
Prep and Cooking Time: 00:15:00

What to Use

- Rolled oats (.5 cup)
- Banana (one, ripe)
- Almond milk (.5 cup or more)
- Almond extract (One tsp)
- Salt (pinch)
- Cinnamon (.25 teaspoon)
- Artificial sweetener (to taste, replaces honey in original recipe)

What to Do

- Cut the banana in half. Mash half of it and put the mashed part into a saucepan.
- Pour the almond milk, almond extract, cinnamon and salt into the saucepan. Stir.
- Bring to a boil, adding more almond milk if needed.
- Simmer 5-7 mins
- Add sweetener to taste.
- Put into serving bowl.
- Dice other half of banana and places slices on top of oatmeal.
- Sprinkle more cinnamon on top if desired.

Pot Roast

Several Servings
Prep and Cooking Time: 04:00:00

What to Use

- Beef chuck (4-5 pounds)
- Healthy fat (as needed)
- Flour (as needed)
- Salt (.5 teaspoon or to taste)
- Horseradish (.5 cup)
- Onions (8-10 small, cut into small pieces)
- Carrots (8-10 small, cut into chunks or sections)
- Celery (8-10 stalks, cut into chunks or sections)
- Potatoes (8-10 peeled, cut into chunks)

What to Do

- Put some flour in a bowl. Season it with salt.
- Roll the beef in the flour mixture to coat all sides.
- Put healthy oil in a kettle and heat it up.
- Put the beef in the hot oil and brown it on all sides.
- Coat with the horseradish.
- Add enough water at the bottom to not burn it.
- Cover and cook slowly for 3-3.5 hours, checking and adding more water if needed.
- During the last hour, cut up and add the vegetables to the roast.

Meat Loaf
Servings: 8
Prep and Cooking Time: 01:40:00

What to Use

- Ground beef (1 pound)
- Lean pork (.5 pound)
- Bread crumbs (2 cups)
- Egg (one, beaten)
- Low-fat milk (1.5 cups)
- Minced onions (4 tablespoons)
- Salt (2 teaspoons)
- Black pepper (.25 teaspoon)
- Dry mustard (.25 teaspoon)
- Sage (.125 teaspoon)
- Sugar-free ketchup (3 tablespoons)

What to Do

- Mix all ingredients together.
- Grease a 9x5x3" loaf pan with healthy oil.
- Pack the meat mixture into the pan.
- Spread ketchup
- Bake for 1.5 hours (350F)

Side Dish Recipes

Pumpkin, Squash, Sweet Potato and Coconut Milk Soup

Several Servings
Prep and Cooking Time: 03:30:00

What to Use
- Pumpkin (1 medium)
- Acorn squash (1 squash)
- Sweet potatoes (2 large)
- Chicken broth (two 14.5-ounce)
- Coconut milk (two 14-ounce)
- Lime (one, juice)
- Ginger (pinch, ground)
- Seasonings (pepper and salt)

What to Do
- Preheat oven to 375 degrees Fahrenheit.
- Puncture pumpkin and squash several times. Wrap the sweet potatoes in aluminum foil. Place all three vegetables onto a baking sheet.
- Bake until pumpkin begins to cave in, around 2 hours.
- Take the skin off of the sweet potatoes, pumpkin and acorn squash.
- Take the seeds out of the the pumpkin and acorn squash.
- Chop and mash (or blend) all three vegetables together until smooth.
- Stir in all but .5 cup of the coconut milk.
- Stir in the chicken broth.
- Mix all the seasonings.
- Cook for few mins (medium heat)
- Dish up. Drizzle coconut milk over the top. Serve with a lime wedge.

Curried Cauliflower and Roasted Carrot Soup

Several Servings
Prep and Cooking Time: 01:10:00

What to Use

- Cauliflower (.5 head, trimmed and chopped)
- Carrots (6 carrots, peeled and chopped)
- Olive oil (1.5 teaspoon)
- Garlic (2 cloves, chopped)
- Pepper and salt (1tsp each)
- Vegetable broth (3 cups or more)
- Curry powder (One tbsp)
- Coconut milk (1 cup)
- Lime (.5 of a lime, juiced)

What to Do

- Mix the cauliflower, carrots, olive oil, garlic, salt and pepper in a casserole dish.
- Roast the mixture in the oven for 20 mins. Stir and roast another 25 mins or until slightly charred. Stir.
- Bring the broth to boil, mix with curry powder and roasted vegetables
- Continue to boil another 8-10 mins or until the vegetables are soft.

Green Pea Salad with Cheddar Cheese
Several Servings
Prep and Cooking Time: 00:15:00

What to Use

- Sweet peas (three 14.5-ounce cans, drained)
- Eggs (three, hard-boiled, cubed)
- Low-fat cheddar cheese (.75 cup, cubed)
- Low-fat mayonnaise (.66 cup)
- Onion (.5 cup, chopped)
- Seasonings (pepper and salt)

What to Do

- Boil the eggs. Let cool then chop them. Put chopped eggs into a large bowl.
- Chop the onion. Add the onions to the bowl with the eggs.
- Cube the cheese. Add the cheese to the bowl.
- Open and drain the cans of peas. Add the peas to the bowl.
- Add the mayonnaise. Mix thoroughly.
- Season to taste.

Veggie-Stuffed Red Bell Peppers

Several Servings
Prep and Cooking Time: 01:00:00

What to Use

- Quinoa (One cup)
- Water (One cup)
- Red bell peppers (two, fresh)
- Granny Smith apple (.5 of apple, cored)
- Lime juice (One tbsp)
- Olive oil (One tsp)
- Minced garlic (One clove)
- Parsley (1.5 tablespoons, fresh)
- Mint (1.5 tablespoons, fresh, chopped)
- Tomatoes (1 cup, chopped)
- Sea salt (to taste)
- Black pepper (to taste)

What to Do

- Boil the quinoa in water for 20-25 mins. Meanwhile, chop the parsley, mint, tomatoes, and the green onions. Place them together in a large bowl.
- Set oven to 350F
- Lightly oil the bottom of a small baking dish.
- Cut the red peppers in half lengthwise. Remove their ribs and seeds, but leave the stems intact. Place peppers cut side up into the baking dish.
- Put the cooked quinoa into the large bowl that contains the chopped vegetables. Mix. Season to taste.
- Stuff the bell pepper halves with the vegetable mixture.
- Optional: Wrap the individual pepper halves containing the mixture with aluminum foil to keep the food moist and to ensure it cooks evenly. Cleanup would also be easier afterwards.
- Fill the bottom of the baking dish with water until the water reaches a depth of .25 inch.
- Bake for 20 mins till the bell peppers are tender.

Snack Recipes

Healthy Banana Pancakes

Servings: 1-2
Prep and Cooking Time: 00:20:00

What to Use

- Eggs (Two)
- Banana (One)
- Oats (.5 cup)
- Apple sauce, unsweetened (.25 cup)
- Vanilla (One tsp)
- Cinnamon (.5 teaspoon)
- Healthy oil (as needed)

What to Do

- Blend oats in Magic Bullet until finely ground.
- Add all the other ingredients and blend until smooth.
- Heat up a healthy oil in the skillet.
- Fry up pancakes.

Cheese Mold with Fruit
Several Servings
Prep Time: 00:20:00

What to Use

- Low-fat cream cheese (one 12-ounce package)
- Low-fat mild American cheese (1 cup, shredded)
- Salt (One tsp)
- Paprika (.5 teaspoon)
- Unflavored gelatin (2 envelopes)
- Water (.5 cup, cold)
- Skim milk (as needed)
- Low-fat Cool Whip (2 cups)
- Healthy oil (as needed to grease mold)
- Fruit (as desired, any kind)

What to Do

- Mix the gelatin with the water. Dissolve over hot water.
- Cream together in a separate bowl the cream cheese, American cheese, salt and paprika.
- Add the dissolved gelatin and the Cool Whip to the bowl. Mix.
- Grease a 9-inch ring gelatin mold with healthy oil.
- Pour the cheesy gelatin mixture into the mold. Chill until set.
- Put lettuce leaves onto a large plate.
- Turn out the gelatin onto the lettuce leaves.
- Garnish the inside and the outside of the gelatin ring with fresh fruit.

Cottage Cheese Egg Salad

Servings: 1-2
Prep and Cooking Time: 00:15:00

What to Use

- Eggs (2 eggs)
- Non-fat cottage cheese (.75 cup, thick, drained)
- Salt (.25 teaspoon)
- Dill, dried (.25 teaspoon)
- Lemon juice (.5 teaspoon)

What to Do

- Boil the eggs. Drain and let cool.
- Finely chop the hard-boiled eggs.
- Drain the non-fat cottage cheese.
- Mix all ingredients together.
- Chill. Note: You won't miss having mayo in this version of the egg salad!

April's Deviled Eggs

Servings: 2-3
Prep and Cooking Time: 00:30:00

What to Use

- Eggs (hard-boiled)
- Prepared mustard (One tbsp)
- Low-fat mayonnaise (One tbsp)
- Garlic salt (.5 teaspoon)
- Onion powder (.5 teaspoon)
- Paprika (pinch)

What to Do

- Boil eggs in a saucepan, covered, for 10-15 mins. Drain the hot water and replace the hot water with cold water a couple of times until the eggs cool.
- Remove shells. Cut in half lengthwise and place into the container you wish to refrigerate them in.
- Remove the yolks and place them into a mixing bowl. Break up into smaller pieces.
- Add the mayonnaise, mustard, garlic salt and the onion powder to the yolks. Mix thoroughly, mashing eggs yolks as you go, until it reaches a smooth consistency.
- Scoop out some of the egg yolk mixture and add it to the egg white.
- Garnish with paprika.
- Cover and refrigerate at least one hour before eating.

Slow Cooker Applesauce

Servings: 6
Prep and Cooking Time: 05:10:00

What to Use

- Sweet red apples (12 Fuji, Honeycrisp or Pink Lady apples)
- Cinnamon (1.5 tablespoons, ground)
- Raisins (.25 cup, optional)

What to Do

- Stem, seed, core the apples. Cut them into chunks. Place the apple chunks into your slow cooker.
- Add the cinnamon and raisins to the apples.
- Cover and cook on high temperature for 4-5 hours, or cook it on low temperature for up to 12 hours. Stir only once during cooking.
- Let cool. Transfer to a container and chill. Eat cold for maximum sweetness.

Dessert Recipes

Cottage Cheese Lemon Fluff
Servings: 8
Prep Time: 00:10:00

What to Use

- Low-fat cottage cheese (3 cups, drained)
- Sugar-free lemon Jell-O (two 0.3-ounce packages, dry mix)
- Cool Whip Lite (one 8-ounce container, thawed)

What to Do

- Blend the cottage cheese in blender until creamy.
- Add the gelatin powder and the whipped cream. Blend until fully mixed.
- Refrigerate. Serve cold.

Peanut Butter-Banana Soft Serve

Servings: 1-2

Prep Time: 00:20:00

What to Use

- Bananas (2 frozen, broken into large pieces)
- Mango (1 cup, frozen, chunks)
- Unsalted peanut butter (2 tablespoons), or use raw almond butter
- Vanilla extract (.5 teaspoon)
- Non-dairy milk (.25 cup)
- Carob powder (One tsp), or cacao powder or cocoa powder

What to Do

- Mix in a food processor (not in a blender). Run until smooth.
- Eat immediately.

Pumpkin Cheesecake

Servings: 8
Prep Time: 00:15:00

What to Use

- Fat-free cream cheese (8-ounce package)
- Pumpkin (1 cup, canned, no salt added)
- Splenda (12 teaspoons)
- Pumpkin pie spice (.5 teaspoon)
- Cool Whip Lite (2 cups, frozen)

What to Do

- Blend the first four ingredients together in a blender.
- Add the Cool Whip. Blend.
- Skip the graham cracker crust and chill.

Fruity, Nutty Jell-O
Several Servings
Prep Time: 00:20:00

What to Use

- Sugar-free Jell-O (1 large package, any flavor, prepared per directions)
- Fruit cocktail (1 small can, unsweetened, drained), or banana (one, cut up)
- Low-fat cream cheese (small block, cut into small chunks), or low-fat sour cream (.5 cup or to taste)
- Pecans or walnuts (.25 cup, chopped extra small; optional and for after your doctor clears you for hard foods)
- Sugar-free Cool Whip (to taste)

What to Do

- Prepare Jell-O per the directions, but don't set up yet.
- Open the can of fruit, drain the juice, and stir the fruit into the Jell-O.
- Cut the cream cheese into chunks and stir the chunks into the Jell-O.
- Add and stir in the nuts (if you are cleared by the doctor for them).
- Let the Jell-O set up.
- Dish up Jell-O into serving bowl. Top with whip topping and more nuts if desired.

Drink Recipes

Peanut Butter-Vanilla Shake

Servings: 1
Prep Time: 00:10:00

What to Use

- Water (8 ounces)
- Vanilla protein powder (2 scoops)
- Vanilla sugar-free instant pudding mix (One tbsp)
- Fruit-flavored sugar-free syrup (One tbsp)
- Creamy low-sugar peanut butter (One tbsp)
- Ice (3-5 cubes)

What to Do

- Blend together all ingredients except for the ice and peanut butter.
- Add ice and blend until slivered.
- Add peanut butter and blend just a few seconds.

Instant-Coffee Frappuccino

Servings: 1
Prep Time: 00:10:00

What to Use

- Skim milk (.5 cup)
- Instant coffee (One tbsp)
- Chocolate or vanilla protein powder (1 scoop)
- Ice (2 handfuls)

What to Do

- Blend all ingredients except for the ice.
- Add ice and blend.

Quick Frappuccino

Servings: 1
Prep Time: 00:10:00

What to Use

- Blue Luna Light Mocha (.5 can, or use a Starbucks Light Frappuccino)
- Chocolate protein powder (1 scoop)

What to Do

- Mix together.
- Put ice in a glass and pour mixture into glass.

Double-Trouble Fudge Shake

Servings: 1
Prep Time: 00:10:00

What to Use

- Water (12 ounces, cold)
- DaVinci sugar-free vanilla syrup (.5 ounce)
- Sugar-free fudgesicle (one)
- Chocolate protein powder (1.5 scoops)
- Splenda (10 packets)
- Ice (6 cubes)

What to Do

- Blend all ingredients together except for the ice and the protein.
- Add and blend the ice one by one.
- Add the protein powder and blend a few seconds on low or medium.

Morning Smoothie
Servings: 2
Prep Time: 00:10:00

What to Use
- Orange juice (.25 cup, fresh squeezed)
- Skim milk (.75 cup)
- Vanilla protein powder (1 scoop)
- Nonfat sugar-free strawberry yogurt (.5 cup)
- Banana (1 small)

What to Do

- Blend and enjoy.

Iced Mocha Latte
Servings: 1
Prep Time: 00:10:00

What to Use
- Cold coffee (to taste, maybe decaf Hazelnut, liquid)
- ProScore 100 chocolate (2 scoops)
- Sugar-free hazelnut coffee syrup (a splash)
- Fat-free, sugar-free vanilla pudding mix (One tbsp)
- Ice (a few cubes)

What to Do

- Blend all together except for the ice.
- Add ice and blend one cube at a time until you reach the desired consistency.

White Chocolate-Coffee Delight
Servings: 1
Prep Time: 00:10:00

What to Use
- ProBlend 55 mocha Cappuccino (1 scoop)
- White chocolate sugar-free syrup (One tbsp)
- Water (splash, ice cold)
- Coffee (splash)

What to Do
- Blend.

Vanilla Pina Colada Shake
Servings: 1
Prep Time: 00:10:00

What to Use
- Vanilla sugar-free pudding mix (2 tablespoons)
- ProScore 100 vanilla (2 scoops)
- Pineapple flavoring (dash)
- Coconut flavoring (dash)
- Ice (few cubes)

What to Do
- Blend all but the ice.
- Add and blend ice cubes one at a time until desired consistency is reached.

Fudge Shake

Servings: 1
Prep Time: 00:10:00

What to Use

- Chocolate fudge sugar-free pudding mix (2 tablespoon)
- ProScore 100 chocolate (2 scoops)
- Water (8 ounces)
- Ice (5 large cubes)

What to Do

- Mix all together except for the ice.
- Blend in the ice, one cube at a time until you reach desired consistency.

Chapter 4: Month Three to Month Six and Beyond

No doubt you have lost a lot of weight after three or so months on your new diet. You are looking good in your new clothes and are receiving a lot of complements. You no longer hurt much either.

You are enjoying food again and have discovered new healthy and tasty recipes that you have tried and love.

You know your stomach is smaller and that what you put in it is important. You need **quality, nutrient-rich food, low-calorie drinks**, and you need to continue to consume small amounts of food and to **drink your 64 ounces of daily fluids** between meals so that you do not stretch your stomach out. You don't want to end up gaining the weight back after all of your hard work, pain, trouble and expense.

Somewhere around month three **your surgeon should give you the okay to start eating solid food**. Hooray!

Included in the new food may be crunchy and spicy food that your system may not tolerate. As always, introduce one new thing at a time and document what your system does not tolerate. You also still need to chew your food well, eat slowly and follow the other guidelines mentioned repeatedly in the former chapters.

Meal Recipes

Southwestern Scrambled Eggs

Protein: 10.62 grams
Calories: 169.8
Servings: 4
Prep and Cooking Time: 00:15:00

What to Use

- Olive oil (One tsp)
- Cilantro (.25 cup, fresh and finely chopped)
- Red onion (.25 cup, chopped)
- Eggs (3 large, with omega 3)
- Non-fat milk (.25 cup, no added vitamin A & D)
- Salt (.5 teaspoon)
- Black pepper (.25, ground)
- Muir Glen Medium Salsa (.5 cup)

What to Do

- Mince the garlic.
- Heat up healthy oil in skillet.
- Add garlic, onion and cilantro.
- Saute five mins or until veggies are soft.
- In a bowl, beat the eggs. Add milk, salt and pepper. Mix together.
- Pour egg mixture into skillet and let cook for two mins, stirring and lifting up the eggs.
- Put eggs onto plate and top with salsa.

Swiss Steak

Servings: 1
Prep and Cooking Time: 01:35:00

What to Use

- Round or flank steak (2 pounds, 1.5 inches thick)
- Cooked tomatoes (#1 tall can)
- Onion (one, sliced)
- Celery (one stalk, diced)
- Flour (as needed to coat steak)
- Salt (as needed to season coating)
- Healthy oil (as needed to brown the steak

What to Do

- Cut up the onion and the celery and set aside.
- Put flour and salt into a bowl and mix together.
- Coat the steak in the flour and salt mixture.
- Heat up oil in heavy skillet.
- Brown the steak on both sides in the hot oil.
- Add the cooked tomatoes and the sliced fresh vegetables to the pan.
- Cover and cook over low heat (or bake in oven set at 300 degrees Fahrenheit) for 2-2.5 hours.

Braised Pork Chops with Sweetened Apple Ring

Servings: 3
Prep and Cooking Time: 01:00:00

What to Use

- Pork chops (one to three, as desired)
- Flour (as needed)
- Salt (as needed)
- Apple (1 fresh, tart, cut into one .75-inch thick slice for each chop)
- Healthy oil (as needed)
- Sugar-free brown sugar (to taste)
- Water (as needed)

What to Do

- Put enough flour, seasoned to taste with salt, to coat the pork chops.
- Heat up healthy oil in an oiled heavy skillet.
- Coat pork chops and place them into the hot skillet. Brown both sides of all chops.
- Place one apple ring on top of each chop. Sprinkle brown sugar on top of the apple rings.
- Add a bit of water to the bottom of the pan. Cover and cook (braise) over low heat for 35-40 mins or until tender.

Chicken Salad

Servings: 6
Prep and Cooking Time: 00:30:00

What to Use

- Chicken (2 cups, cooked, chopped, cold)
- Eggs (2-3 eggs, hard-boiled, chopped, cold; one could be reserved for presentation)
- Celery (1 cup, fresh)
- Lemon juice (One tbsp)
- Seasonings (pepper and salt)
- Low-fat mayonnaise (.5 cup)
- Tomato (one, fresh, optional)
- Lettuce (optional)
- Olives (optional)
- Sweet pickles (optional)
- Parsley (optional)

What to Do

- Bake, cool and chop the chicken.
- Boil, cool and chop the eggs that will be mixed with the chicken.
- Chop the celery.
- Put the chicken, celery, lemon juice, salt and pepper in a bowl. Mix.
- Add and mix in the mayonnaise.
- Add and mix in the chopped eggs.
- Optional presentation:
- Cover bottom of plate with lettuce leaves.
- Cut the tomato downward from the top, but not through the bottom, between two and four times so as to make a tomato flower cup for the salad.
- Put the tomato flower on top of the lettuce and fill with the chicken.
- Top the chicken with fresh parsley.
- Slice the remaining boiled egg into slices.
- Line the edge of the flower with the egg slices, olives, sweet pickles, etc., as desired.

Side Dish Recipes

Cabbage Salad

Servings: 4
Prep Time: 00:10

What to Use

- Cabbage (2.5 cups, shredded)
- Salt (One tsp)
- Low-fat mayonnaise (as needed to coat)

What to Do

- Mix all ingredients together.

Potato Salad
Servings:6
Prep Time: 02:20:00

What to Use

- Potatoes (3 cups, cubed, boiled, cold)
- Onion (One tbsp, finely chopped)
- Salt (dash)
- Black pepper (dash)
- Pimiento (to taste, optional)
- Parsley (to taste, optional)
- French dressing (.25 cup)
- Low-fat mayonnaise (.75 cup)

What to Do

- Boil the eggs. Let cool. Chill.
- Peel, cube, boil the potatoes until soft but not falling apart. Cool.
- Chop the onions.
- Put the cooled potatoes and the onions together in a bowl.
- Season with salt and pepper. Mix gently.
- Add the French dressing. Mix gently. Chill 1-2 hours.
- Add the mayonnaise, pimiento and parsley. Mix gently.
- Dice and add the chilled eggs. Mix gently.
- Add extra seasonings to taste.
- Dish up into individual bowls. For more variety, place on individual plates surrounded with salad greens, cucumber sticks, slices of boiled eggs, and/or tomato sections.

Indian-Style Rice with Raisins, Cashews and Turmeric

Servings: 3-6
Prep and Cooking Time: 00:30:00

- Note: Ask your doctor whether you can have this much starch.

What to Use
- Basmati rice (1.5 cups, uncooked)
- Coconut milk (one 14-ounce can)
- Chicken stock (14 ounces)
- Olive oil (One tbsp, any healthy oil)
- Cumin (.5 teaspoon)
- Coriander (.5 teaspoon, ground)
- Red pepper flakes (1 pinch, crushed)
- Salt (One tsp)
- Turmeric (.25 teaspoon, ground)
- Raisins (.5 cup)
- Cashew halves (.75 cup)
- Bay leaf (one, fresh)

What to Do
- Heat oil in a large saucepan over medium-high heat.
- Stir in the uncooked rice. Cook for 2 mins.
- Pour in the chicken stock, coconut milk, cumin, coriander, turmeric, red pepper flakes, salt, bay leaf, raisins, and cashew nuts.
- Bring to a boil, then reduce the heat to low. Cover and cook for about 20 mins or until the rice is tender.
- If you want a decorative presentation, press the rice mixture into a lightly oiled bowl, invert and unmold onto serving plate. Then put lime slices around the base. Put extra cashews and raisins around the sides. Garnish the top with fresh chopped tomato, fresh cilantro.

Snack Recipes

Raw Veggies with Hummus Dip
Several Servings
Prep Time: 00:20:00

What to Use

- Garbanzo beans (2 cups, canned, drained)
- Garlic (2 cloves, halved)
- Lemon juice (.25 cup)
- Tahini (.33 cup)
- Salt (One tsp)
- Olive oil (One tbsp)
- Paprika (pinch)
- Parsley (handful, fresh, chopped)
- Raw veggies (amount as needed)

What to Do

- Blend the first five ingredients together.
- Transfer mixture into a bowl.
- Drizzle the olive oil on top. Sprinkle with paprika. Sprinkle chopped, fresh parsley on top.
- Dip boiled or steamed carrots in hummus.

Tuna Cucumber Snack

Several Servings

Prep Time: 00:20:00

What to Use

- Cucumbers (one or two)
- Tuna (1 small can, packed in water, drained)
- Low-fat mayonnaise (.5 cup)
- Peas (.5 can), or carrots (.5 can), or corn (.5 can)
- Salt (to taste)
- Black pepper (to taste)

What to Do

- Mix together the tuna, peas and the mayonnaise in a bowl.
- Take the skins off of the cucumber(s). Slice the cucumber(s) into sections one inch wide.
- Core out a "bowl" in the seed area of each cucumber with a melon baller or spoon. Lay cucumber sections down into a (preferable sealable) container, bowl side up.
- Fill the tiny cucumber bowls with the tuna mixture.
- Cover and keep refrigerated.

Ants on a Log (Cream Cheese-Filled Celery)
Several Servings
Prep Time: 00:20:00

What to Use

- Celery (one or more stalks, as desired)
- Low-fat cream cheese (one small block)
- Raisins (as needed)

What to Do

- Break off celery stalk(s) desired. Wash off the dirt.
- Cut celery into sections two to three inches long.
- Fill celery sections with cream cheese.
- Put raisins in the cheese, down the middle of each section.
- Put into a container, covered. Keep refrigerated.

Baked Kale Chips

Several Servings
Prep and Cooking Time: 00:30:00

What to Use

- Kale (1 bunch, fresh)
- Olive oil (One tbsp)
- Seasoned salt (One tsp)

What to Do

- Preheat oven to 350 degrees Fahrenheit.
- Line a cookie sheet with parchment paper.
- Cut the kale leaves from off the stems.
- Wash the kale leaves. Dry them thoroughly.
- Tear the leaves into bite-size pieces.
- Add the oil and thoroughly coat the leaves.
- Lay the leaves out on the baking sheet
- Sprinkle the leaves with the seasoning salt.
- Bake 10-15 mins or until the edges are brown but not burned.
- Dip into hummus or another healthy dip.

Watermelon Salsa
Several Servings
Prep Time: 00:20:00

What to Use

- Watermelon (8 cups, seeded, cubed)
- Cilantro (1 bunch, fresh, chopped)
- White onion (.5 large, chopped)
- Jalapeno peppers (2 large, stemmed, seeded, and minced)
- Garlic (2 cloves, minced)
- White wine vinegar (1 cup)
- Salt (One tsp)

What to Do

- Cut up, seed and measure the watermelon. Put it into a large bowl.
- Chop and measure the onion. Add the chopped onion to the bowl with the watermelon.
- Stem, seed and mince the jalapeno peppers. Add the minced peppers to the bowl.
- Mince the garlic cloves. Add the minced garlic to the bowl.
- Add the vinegar to the mixture. Mix well.
- Season with the salt to taste.
- Cover and chill overnight.
- Dip kale chips or other healthy snack food in it.

Healthy Peanut Butter Cookies
Several Servings
Prep and Cooking Time: 00:15:00

What to Use

- Natural peanut butter (2 cups, smooth)
- Eggs (2 large)
- Splenda (2 cups granular)

What to Do

- Preheat oven to 350 degrees Fahrenheit.
- Beat the eggs in a large mixing bowl
- Add the Splenda and then the peanut butter.
- Thoroughly mix the ingredients together.
- Drop by spoonfuls onto baking sheet.
- Bake about 8 mins.

Cinnamon Vanilla Granola

Several Servings
Prep and Cooking Time: 01:30:00

What to Use

- Old-fashioned oats (3 cups)
- Quick oats (2 cups)
- Pecans (1 cup, chopped), or almonds (1 cup, sliced), or sunflower seeds (1 cup)
- Wheat germ (.5 cup, toasted)
- Real maple syrup (.25 cup)
- Healthy oil (2 tablespoons)
- Vanilla extract (2 tablespoons)
- Cinnamon (4 teaspoons, ground)
- Nutmeg (.5 teaspoon)
- Dried cranberries (1 cup), or raisins (1 cup), or other dried fruit (1 cup)

What to Do

- Mix together the old-fashioned oats, the quick oats, wheat germ and pecans in a large bowl.
- In a small bowl, mix together the maple syrup, oil, nutmeg, cinnamon and vanilla.
- Pour the contents of the small bowl into the large bowl. Mix all ingredients together thoroughly.
- Grease a baking sheet with healthy oil.
- Coat the granola mixture out evenly over the sheet.
- Bake at 300 degrees Fahrenheit for 50-60 mins, taking them out and stirring them every 15 mins. Bake until the oats are toasted.
- Remove sheet from oven.
- Put into a pan and stir in the dried fruit.
- Cool on a wire rack.
- Then transfer to and store in an airtight container.
- Use to top yogurt, fresh fruit, etc.

Dessert Recipes

Peanut Butter Chocolate Pudding
Servings: 4
Prep Time: 00:10:00

What to Use

- Natural peanut butter (.25 cup)
- Cocoa powder (2 tablespoons, natural)
- Unsweetened almond milk (.25 cup)
- Avocado (1 ripe Haas)
- Banana (1 ripe, medium-sized)
- Medjool dates (8, pitted)
- Cacao nibs (One tsp, optional)
- Peanuts (One tsp, optional)

What to Do

- Blend together the almond milk, dates, cocoa powder, peanut butter, avocado, and banana in a blender on high setting for 30 seconds or until completely blended.
- Put into individual serving bowls.
- Top with cacao nibs and/or peanuts if desired.
- Refrigerate up to three days.

Raw Chocolate-Orange-Hemp Bites

Servings: 15
Prep Time: 00:15:00

What to Use

- Organic unsulfured dates (1 cup, pitted)
- Organic Ceylon cinnamon (.5 teaspoon, ground)
- Organic orange flavor (.125 teaspoon)
- Vitamin C powder (1 scoop, made from whole foods)
- Organic cocoa powder (2 tablespoons)
- Organic extra virgin coconut oil (One tbsp)
- Organic coconut flakes (.25 cup, unsweetened, dried)
- Organic hemp seeds (.5 cup)
- Organic almonds (1.5 cups, preferably soaked, rinsed and dehydrated)

What to Do

- Optional: Soak the almonds in a bowl full of filtered water overnight. Place the soaked almonds on a flat tray and dehydrate for 12-14 hours at 115 degrees Fahrenheit or until completely dry.
- Blend together in a food processor the cinnamon, orange extract, vitamin C powder, cocoa powder, coconut oil, coconut flakes, hemp seeds and the almonds for about 30 seconds.
- Set the food processor to high and feed it the dates one by one. Run the processor for 2 mins or until the ingredients start to form a ball. Stop and scrape down the sides.
- Form 12-15 "cookies" with your (washed) hands, and place them in container for refrigerator.
- Chill.

Date-Hemp Energy Balls

Servings:12
Prep and Cooking Time: 00:50:00

What to Use

- Medjool dates (10 large, pitted)
- Pumpkins seeds (1 cup)
- Hemp seeds (.25 cup)
- Vanilla extract (.5 teaspoon)
- Coconut oil (One tbsp)
- Coconut flour (2 tablespoons)
- Carob or cocoa powder (One tsp)
- Shredded coconut (2 tablespoons, toasted, optional)

What to Do

- Put all ingredients except for the shredded coconut into a food processor. Pulse for 45 seconds.
- Pour into a medium mixing bowl.
- Use your (washed) hands to form 12 balls, rolling each ball over a plate of shredded coconut, if desired, and placing into refrigerator container.
- Chill at least 30 mins.

Berry Crumbs

Servings: 4
Prep and Cooking Time: 01:10:00

What to Use
- Strawberries (2 cups, fresh or frozen)
- Blueberries (1.5 cups, fresh or frozen)
- Lemon juice (One tsp)
- Vanilla extract (.5 teaspoon)
- Cassava flour (.5 cup), or oat flour or other flour
- Coconut flour (2 tablespoons)
- Coconut sugar (2 tablespoons), or substitute
- Baking powder (.25 teaspoon)
- Seas salt (pinch)
- Coconut oil (2 tablespoons, melted)

What to Do
- Defrost frozen berries.
- Preheat oven to 350 degrees Fahrenheit.
- Lightly grease 8 x 8-inch glass baking dish with healthy oil. Set aside.
- In a bowl, stir to mix the vanilla extract, lemon juice, strawberries and blueberries. Pour mixture into prepared baking dish.
- In a medium bowl, combine the sea salt, baking powder, coconut oil, coconut sugar, coconut flour and cassava flour. Use your (washed) hands, if necessary, to assure it becomes crumbly.
- Drop by tablespoons on top of the berry mixture. Coat it out evenly.
- Bake for 45 mins or until crumble topping starts to brown.
- Remove from oven. Let cool 10 or more mins before eating.
- Optional: For added creaminess, you could eat this with a dairy-free milk, yogurt or ice cream.

Dairy-Free Strawberry Ice Cream

Servings:6
Prep Time: 00:30:00

What to Use

- Coconut milk (one 13.5-ounce can, full fat)
- Almond milk (1 cup)
- Medjool dates (1 cup, pitted)
- Strawberries (1 pint)
- Vanilla extract (One tsp)
- Vanilla bean (one)

What to Do

- Chill the can of coconut until fully chilled through.
- In a high-speed blender, mix the almond milk, coconut milk, strawberries, dates, vanilla extract and the vanilla bean seeds on high speed until smooth.
- Pour the blended mixture into the base of the ice cream maker. Process into ice cream.
- Transfer to a container and store the ice cream in your freezer.

Dairy-Free Chocolate-Raspberry Ice Cream

Servings: 1 pint
Prep Time: 01:10:00

What to Use

- Coconut milk (one 13.5-ounce can, full fat, chilled)
- Raspberries (1 pint, fresh, or 1 cup frozen and defrosted)
- Medjool dates (1 cup = about 12 large dates, pitted)
- Cocoa powder (.25 cup)
- Vanilla extract (.5 teaspoon)
- Fresh mint leaves (6-8 leaves)

What to Do

- Freeze the bottom of your ice cream maker.
- Chill the can of coconut milk.
- Put the coconut milk, vanilla, cocoa powder, and raspberries in a food processor. Process on high until combined.
- Pour the mixture into the base of the ice cream maker. Churn for 30 mins.
- Transfer the ice cream to a glass container. Freeze in your freezer for at least 30 mins. Tastes best if eaten on during the same day it was made.

Dairy-Free Sweet Cherry Ice Cream

Servings: 6
Prep Time: 00:30:00

What to Use

- Cherries (two 10-ounce bags, one bag frozen and one bag defrosted in refrigerator)
- Coconut milk (one 13.5-ounce can, full-fat, chilled)
- Vanilla extract (2 teaspoons)
- Carob powder (2 tablespoons)
- Medjool dates (1.5 cups = 12 dates)
- Soy milk (1.25 cups, unsweetened), or your favorite non-dairy milk

What to Do

- Blend all ingredients *except for the defrosted bag of cherries* in a high-speed blender until smooth.
- Taste and add more dates if more sweetness is desired.
- Put the blended mixture into the base of an ice cream maker. Process until frozen.
- Serve with a scoop of the defrosted cherries on top.
- Keep the ice cream frozen in your freezer.

Drink Recipes

Peanut-Banana-Chocolate Shake

Servings:2
Prep Time: 00:10:00

What to Use

- Almond milk (.5 cup, unsweetened)
- Chocolate protein powder (1 scoop)
- Vanilla extract (2 teaspoon)
- PB2 (One tbsp, regular or chocolate)
- Banana (.5 of banana, frozen)
- Ice (4-5 cubes)

What to Do

- Blend all ingredients except for the ice.
- Add ice one cube at a time until blended and desired consistency is reached.

Orange-Banana Morning

Servings: 2
Prep Time: 00:10:00

What to Use

- Water (.5 cup, cold)
- Orange juice (.5 cup, no pulp)
- Banana (.5 of banana, sliced)
- Keto Shake Banana Crème protein powder (1 scoop)
- Keto Shake Orange Crème protein powder (1 scoop)
- Ice (1 cup)

What to Do

- Blend all except for the ice.
- Add and blend ice cubes one at a time until you reach the desired consistency.

Ultimate Orange Julius Smoothie
Serving:1
Prep Time: 00:10:00

What to Use

- Water (6 ounces)
- Orange juice (.25 cup, preferably fresh squeezed)
- Vanilla flavoring (One tsp)
- ProScore 100 vanilla (2 scoops)
- Sugar-free vanilla pudding mix (One tbsp)
- Ice (3-4 cubes)

What to Do

- Blend all ingredients except for the ice.
- Add and blend ice cubes one at a time until you reach the desired consistency.

Campfire Delight Shake

Serving:1
Prep Time: 00:10:00

What to Use

- Sans Sucre Cinnamon-Sugar (to taste)
- Vitamite (a splash)
- DaVinci Sugar-Free Toasted Marshmallow Syrup (to taste)
- ProV60 Chocolate Thunder protein powder (1 scoop)
- Coffee (to taste, optional)
- Ice (a few cubes)

What to Do

- Blend all ingredients together except for the ice.
- Add and blend ice one cube at a time until the you reach the desired consistency.

Creamy Peach
Serving:1
Prep Time: 00:10:00

What to Use

- Sugar-free instant vanilla pudding (2 tablespoons)
- Vanilla protein powder (1 scoop)
- Splenda (6 packets)
- Crystal Lite Peach Tea (6 ounces)
- Ice (few cubes)

What to Do

- Blend all except ice.
- Add and blend ice cubes one at a time until you reach the desired consistency.

Ultimate Chocolate-Banana Protein Shake

Servings:1-2

Prep Time: 00:10:00

What to Use

- Non-fat milk (.5 cup)
- Banana (.5 cup, sliced ripe)
- Banana fat-free sugar-free yogurt (.5 cup)
- Chocolate protein powder (1 scoop)
- Vanilla extract (dash)

What to Do

- Blend, pour into glass and enjoy!

Snicker-Coffee Shake

Serving: 1
Prep Time: 00:10:00

What to Use

- Water (a splash)
- Vitamite (a splash)
- Snickerdoodle Coffee (a splash), or sugar-free hazelnut syrup and sugar-free cinnamon-sugar
- Chocolate protein powder (1 scoop)
- Ice (a few cubes)

What to Do

- Blend all except for the ice.
- Add and blend in ice one cube at a time until you reach the desired consistency.

Candy Bar Shake

Serving: 1
Prep Time: 00:10:00

What to Use

- Water (a splash)
- Chocolate caramel coffee (splash), or regular coffee, sugar-free caramel syrup, or sugar-free chocolate syrup
- Chocolate protein powder (to taste)
- Vitamite (splash)
- Creamy peanut butter (One tsp), or sugar-free peanut butter syrup
- Ice (a few cubes)

What to Do

- Blend all ingredients except for the ice.
- Add and blend ice one cube at a time until you reach the desired consistency.

Cherry-Banana-Chocolate Delight

Serving: 1
Prep Time: 00:10:00

What to Use

- Banana (.5 of banana)
- Maraschino cherries (4 cherries)
- Chocolate Isopure (1 scoop)
- 1% milk (.5 cup)
- Sugar-free chocolate syrup (a splash)
- Ice (1 cup)

What to Do

- Blend all ingredients except for the ice.
- Add and blend ice one cube at a time until you reach the desired consistency.

Spinach and Peanut Butter Shake

Servings: 2
Prep Time: 00:10:00

What to Use

- Almond milk (1 cup, unsweetened)
- Banana (.33 of banana, frozen)
- PB2 or peanut butter (2 tablespoons)
- Vanilla protein powder (1 scoop)
- Coffee (.5 cup, cold)
- Spinach (3 handfuls, fresh)

What to Do

- Blend and enjoy!

Strawberry-Chocolate Milk

Servings: 2
Prep Time: 00:10:00

What to Use

- Water (14 ounces)
- Carb Solutions (1 scoop)
- Strawberry Carb Solutions (2 scoops)
- Carnation Fat-Free Hot Cocoa (1 package)

What to Do

- Blend.

Multi-Berry Delight

Servings: 2
Prep Time: 00:10:00

What to Use

- Cranberry juice (1 cup)
- Blueberries (.25 cup)
- Strawberries (4 berries, frozen or fresh)
- Strawberry Pro Blend 55 (1 scoop)
- Ice (1 cup)

What to Do

- Blend all ingredients except for the ice.
- Add and blend in ice a little at a time until you reach the desired consistency.

Pina Colada

Serving: 1
Prep Time: 00:10:00

What to Use

- Crushed pineapple in unsweetened juice (one 8-ounce can, cold)
- Artificial sweetener (1 packet)
- Coconut extract (One tbsp)
- Vanilla protein powder (1 scoop)
- Ice (.5 cup)

What to Do

- Blend all except for the ice.
- Add and blend ice a little at a time until you reach the desired consistency.

Conclusion

Thank you again for downloading this book!

I hope this book is able to help you as you go through your journey of recovery and on to a thinner, healthier new you.

If your surgery will not take place for another several weeks, you have the advantage of trying out some of the protein drink and other recipes now. You can decide which ones you like best and then stock up on most of the ingredients for them. The fewer trips to the store you or a helper have to make after your surgery, the happier everyone will be.

You will be drinking a lot of protein shakes and protein smoothies during your recovery because they pack a lot of protein in a small amount of drink, and you need to consume a lot of protein during your recovery.

On the other hand, if you just had your gastric sleeve surgery, the next step is to see how these recipe ingredients line up with what your doctor prescribed for you. They should be very closely aligned. If an ingredient is not yet allowed, do what your doctor tells you for each stage of your recovery. You can always wait to try a recipe out after your doctor clears you for that ingredient.

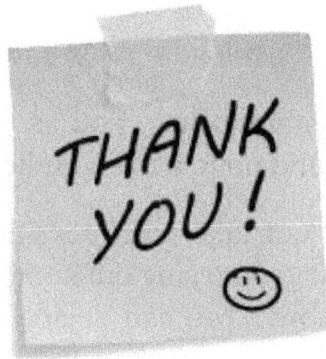

Finally, if you enjoyed this book, then I'd like to ask you for a favor. Would you be kind enough to leave a review for this book on Amazon? It would be greatly appreciated!

Thank you and good luck!

Check Out My Other Books

Below you'll find some of my other popular books that are popular on Amazon and Kindle as well. Simply click on the links below to check them out. Alternatively, you can visit my author page on Amazon to see other work done by me.

CrossFit: Barbell and Dumbbell Exercises for Body Strength

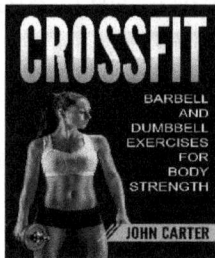

Mediterranean Diet: Step By Step Guide And Proven Recipes For Smart Eating And Weight Loss

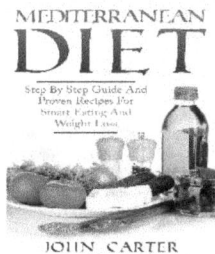

Weight Watchers: Smart Points Cookbook - Step By Step Guide And Proven Recipes For Effective Weight Loss

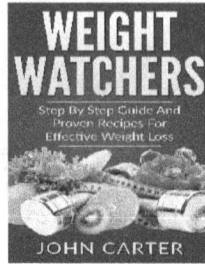

Bodybuilding: Beginners Handbook - Proven Step By Step Guide To Get The Body You Always Dreamed About

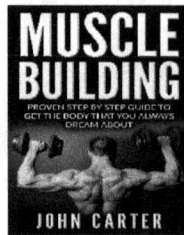

South Beach Diet: Lose Weight and Get Healthy the South Beach Way

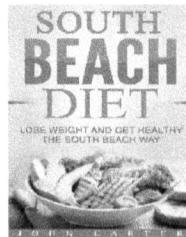

Blood Pressure: Step By Step Guide And Proven Recipes To Lower Your Blood Pressure Without Any Medication

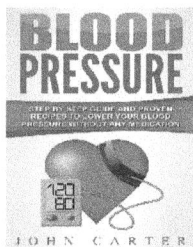

Ketogenic Diet: Step By Step Guide And 70+ Low Carb, Proven Recipes For Rapid Weight Loss

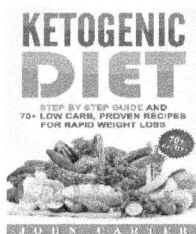

Meal Prep: 65+ Meal Prep Recipes Cookbook – Step By Step Meal Prepping Guide For Rapid Weight Loss

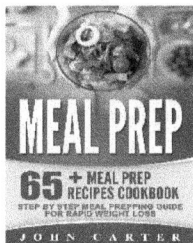

If the links do not work, for whatever reason, you can simply search for these titles on the Amazon website to find them.

www.ingramcontent.com/pod-product-compliance
Lightning Source LLC
Chambersburg PA
CBHW051713020426
42333CB00014B/959